MORE PRAISE FOR ROB GORE

"Dr. Gore's book should be mandatory reading for incoming medical practitioners, law enforcement actors, urban policy professionals, and, most importantly, high school students who are trying to find themselves in generationally hurt communities…. He addresses race, poverty, and trauma with the ease and eloquence of your neighborhood sage. This book is a gift and should be used as a primary surgical tool to treating violence."
—MARLON PETERSON, author of *Bird Uncaged:
An Abolitionist's Freedom Song*

"This book is a moving testament to the enduring power of compassion and the profound impact one person can have on the lives of many. Dr. Rob Gore's story is an inspiring call to action, a reminder that in the face of adversity and violence, there is always hope and there is always a way to make a positive difference."
—DR. NADIA LOPEZ, EdD, author of *The Bridge to Brilliance:
How One Principal in a Tough Community Is Inspiring the World*

"Just what we need to help combat the trauma that ravages emergency departments across the country, as well as the growing epidemic of workplace violence. The impact on our healthcare system and communities is tremendous. Key solutions—education and engagement—are outlined in this book."
—AISHA TERRY, MD, president, American
College of Emergency Physicians

"Few community changemakers use as direct an approach to interrupting violence for our youth as Dr. Rob Gore. His deep commitment to healing trauma and addressing social and environmental causes of community decay has literally and figuratively saved many lives, in plain sight. Many, from the affected youth to our elected leaders, can follow Dr. Gore's lead on ensuring a more equitable and positive future for all."
—SEAN RICE, principal, High School for Public Service

"As we address the critical issue of violence in our communities, Dr. Rob Gore's new book amplifies the need to treat violence as a public health issue while providing tactical and transformative practices that can be implemented across the country. This text should be a part of any city or community focused on truly addressing violence with proven interventions and solutions."
—CHRISTINA GRANT, EdD, superintendent of schools,
Washington, DC

"A deeply personal and wildly eye-opening recollection of daily violence unleashed onto Black bodies through the decades from an author who teetered on both sides of being a person subjugated to these acts and a healer both in the emergency department and global communities. The commonality of these events is a testament to an amalgamation of larger societal issues that BIPOC communities have to constantly grapple with."
—HANK WILLIS THOMAS, conceptual artist, author, and US Department of State Medal of Arts recipient

"Violence is one of the most, if not the most, preventable public health epidemics in our country. As an emergency room physician, Dr. Gore has helped save countless individual victims and has decided to take it a step further to help save communities. His dedication, advocacy, and experience are an inspiration to anyone interested in truly addressing the uniquely American crisis."
—JUMAANE D. WILLIAMS, Public Advocate of the City of New York

"Filled with compelling stories that highlight the horrific epidemic of violence in the US, this book also provides solutions, and not just band-aids for the symptoms but real solutions that deal with the root causes of trauma linked to systemic racism. The book is a wake-up call for all Americans to open our hearts to stop the cycle of violence by allowing people to heal and by stopping the cycle of racism that is rooted so deeply in our nation."
—JEAN OELWANG, CEO of Virgin Unite and author of *Partnering*

"Dr. Rob Gore delves into the somber reality of violence within American society. This gripping book takes readers on a thought-provoking journey, examining violence through the lens of public health while uncovering the harrowing stories of victims and survivors. With its compelling narrative and expert analysis, it is a must-read for anyone seeking to understand and confront the deadly American epidemic of violence."
—ALLISON BRASHEAR, MD, MPH, dean of the Jacobs School of Medicine and Biomedical Sciences, University at Buffalo

"Dr. Gore pulls us into his extraordinary personal journey as a young Black doctor in Brooklyn who vows to stop the trauma of violence before witnessing another person from his community fighting for their life in an emergency room. Gore's sincere love for the people he treats is a healing balm inside these pages and a deliberate call to action that could forever change the way we see and treat violence at its roots."
—JESSICA CARE MOORE, author of *We Want Our Bodies Back*

TREATING VIOLENCE

TREATING VIOLENCE

An Emergency Room Doctor Takes On a Deadly American Epidemic

ROB GORE, MD

BEACON PRESS
BOSTON

BEACON PRESS
Boston, Massachusetts
www.beacon.org

Beacon Press books
are published under the auspices of
the Unitarian Universalist Association of Congregations.

26 25 24   8 7 6 5 4 3 2 1

Some of the names in this book have been changed to protect
identities; the vast majority have not been changed.

This book is printed on acid-free paper that meets the uncoated
paper ANSI/NISO specifications for permanence as revised
in 1992.

Composition by Kevin Barrett Kane at
Wilsted & Taylor Publishing Services

Library of Congress Cataloguing-in-Publication
Data is available for this title.

Hardcover ISBN: 978-0-8070-2016-6

E-book ISBN: 978-0-8070-2019-7

Audiobook: 978-0-8070-0378-7

CONTENTS

INTRODUCTION

CONFRONTING VIOLENCE

I'VE BEEN A PHYSICIAN for over twenty years and my specialty is emergency medicine. For the past sixteen years I have been practicing at both Kings County Hospital and SUNY Downstate Medical Center in the East Flatbush section of Brooklyn, directly across the street from my old elementary school and a twenty- to thirty-minute drive from the Fort Greene neighborhood where I grew up. (I actually grew up in both Fort Greene and Flatbush.) You all will think of the place I work as the ER, for emergency room, but for years now it's been called the ED, for emergency department, in most hospitals.

Occasionally the ED is pretty calm, undramatic. The patients we see present with a wide range of illnesses, diseases, and trauma, both imaginable and unimaginable. Where I practice, the major- ity of what I see is characteristic of underdeveloped and impov- erished communities: the aftermath of systemic racism; the ills of inadequate diets; difficult living conditions; scattered, inconsistent health care for issues like diabetes, asthma, high blood pressure, heart issues; and sometimes just the bumps and bruises of life. And then there are the days, most days, that aren't so quiet. These days are further complicated by shootings, stabbings, rape, other forms of sexual violence, and intimate partner violence, which I see much

I

too often. Usually, the person I'm treating with a fist, knife, or bullet wound is a Black man. When I was a younger physician, my patients and I were often the same age, same style, maybe even from the same area. Even now, as an older physician, the patients are sometimes my age, and from my neighborhood. The motif is common: a Black man losing his life while I am fighting to save it. The cycle is exhausting—and one that needs to end.

In 2016, I was privileged to be chosen as an inaugural member of the TED residency program, which ended in 2019 and was an incubator for people to expand ideas or develop new ones. I had applied, never imagining I would be chosen. Over the fourteen weeks of the residency, I met amazing thinkers and doers of all kinds. It was especially exhilarating to meet and work with people outside the medical profession, people who were developing ideas about everything from ocean conservation to ending mass incarceration. As part of the residency, we were all invited to give a TED Talk and were coached in how to write and deliver it. I had been doing public speaking regularly since high school, but TED Talks have some different aspects, including standing in front of a camera and speaking to a more global and diverse audience. When it was my turn to speak, I began with this story:

> I distinctly remember that he was young, Black, and he looked like me. He was covered in blood the same as me, but the difference was that he was a patient laid out on a stretcher after being shot in the face and chest, and I was the physician who pronounced him dead. He was killed by another young man that looked like him who was also being treated for gunshot wounds in the room next door. Coincidentally, the perpetrator had been shot two years prior by the dead man.[1]

The sad fact is that, according to the Centers for Disease Control, homicide (assault) is the number-two cause of death for Black males ages one to nine and the number-one cause of death for Black men ages fifteen to thirty-four.[2] This means that we are more likely to die at the hands of another person than from cancer or car accidents.

A perfect circle of violence. And one I've committed to disrupting. I do it every day as a doctor; I do it in working with young people through Kings Against Violence Initiative (KAVI), the nonprofit organization I founded that works both to reach young people before they've been victims or perpetrators of violence and to support victims of violence as well as heading off retaliatory violence. And now I'm doing it through this book. I'm hoping to persuade everyone who reads it to join me in the fight to expand the paradigm in the way we approach violence in this country.

Despite New York City's significant reductions in crime and violence over the last thirty years, city safety still leaves much to be desired. In 2021, there were over 1,400 shooting incidents in our city.[3] In fact, homicide is a leading cause of death for fifteen- to twenty-four-year-olds in the city.[4] My home borough of Brooklyn—population 2.7 million—leads the other four boroughs in the number of shootings and violent crimes.[5] Although patients come from all over the city, and all over the world, to be treated where I work, at Kings County Hospital, the majority of patients live in Brooklyn and come from the neighborhoods Flatbush, East Flatbush, Crown Heights, Flatlands, East New York, Canarsie, Bedford-Stuyvesant (also called Bed-Stuy), and Brownsville. The majority of people living in these communities, give or take gentrified members, are Black (Black families who migrated from the southern US, the Caribbean, and/or Africa). Some of these neighborhoods have some of the highest poverty rates in New York City and in the nation. Brownsville, Crown Heights, and East New York have higher percentages of people living in poverty than the rest of New York City.[6] These neighborhoods, in addition to East Flatbush, also have higher rates of violence- and assault-related hospitalizations compared to the rest of the city.[7]

The image of violence in the inner city is one that pervades our culture—on TV shows, in movies, and all over social media; it's deep in the popular imagination as well, but the fact is this is real. We live in a violent society. America is at war with itself. Consider these statistics. More than seven hundred thousand youth between the ages of ten and twenty-four are treated for non-fatal violent injuries in EDs in US hospitals.[8] People injured due to intentional violence are more likely to die from their injuries than people injured due to an accident.[9] Out of all the homicides committed in the US in 2020, 79 percent were by firearms.[10] Many people injured due to intentional violence return to the hospital with repeat injuries. Recidivism is as high as 58 percent within five years after the initial injury, and the mortality rate is as high as 20 percent within five years of the initial injury.[11]

Some of these intentional acts of violence are related to petty crime, some to vengeance, some to hatred, but the result is the same. Lives cut short, families left bereft, a society eroding at its seams. And how do we react? We lock people up. We look away from the trauma and leave traumatized victims and perpetrators to work it out for themselves. All too often, the cycle begins anew.

I am part of a movement with many others all over the country, working toward a different way. What if we treated violence like a contagion, a public health threat, one that can be "treated" in stages? Below is an excerpt taken from one of KAVI's grant proposals:

We believe it's essential to identify trauma first, as a way to get to the root cause of violence, and not just the cause of one presenting violent incident. We begin by recognizing and identifying the trauma has occurred; then we work to determine what is important for those impacted by a violent traumatic event to ensure their short-term and long-term survivability. We are actively seeking to prevent retaliatory violence from occurring, and cultivating safe spaces within the community, free from violence. In the immediate aftermath of violence, we are trying to control and prevent more violence, in the long term the goal is to eradicate interpersonal youth violence.

Here's what we hope to do:
1. Create a space where youth know they have alternatives to violence.

2. Be a resource to youth and to community organizations.
3. Create a template for the program that is sustainable and replicable.
4. Decrease violence rates.
5. Decrease incarceration rates.
6. Increase graduation rates.
7. Increase personal and professional opportunities for youth who are most at risk of being subjected to violence, or possibly of committing violent acts.

In treating disease, illness, trauma, and violence, it is imperative to also seek to understand the cause of these problems, understanding them through a public health lens. The CDC promotes a four-step process (developed over years through the work of many grassroots, community-based organizations, governmental and nongovernmental agencies from around the world) to begin to do that:

1. Define and monitor the problem.
2. Identify risk and protective factors.
3. Develop and test prevention strategies.
4. Assure widespread adoption.[12]

I believe this is the only way to effectively transform the impact of violence, and it's why I started KAVI and remain so committed to its mission. Treating and approaching violence as a public health problem like any other epidemic—crack cocaine, narcotics, and even COVID—understanding the risk factors of violence, identifying who it impacts and how it permeates communities, and mitigating the risk factors can ultimately eradicate it or at least reduce its most harmful impacts.

Rather than locking people up, containing them in communities with minimal resources and limited support, let's treat the trauma and provide alternatives and, above all, head off violence before it even happens.

The chapters of this book correspond to my journey to this con-clusion. The first part of the book covers my life, including my early encounters with violence and my journey to becoming a physician; the second part details the creation of KAVI and shares stories of what we've accomplished. I conclude with some thoughts about how the nation might move forward toward a society that addresses violence in a way that will lead to significant reduction, not just reaction.

I'm not alone in this effort, and KAVI is far from the only pro-gram to address violence; I've learned from and have been inspired by so many and I'll make note of the work nationwide.

I've seen too many people suffer and die at the hands of another human being. I've made it my mission to help stem the tide.

CHAPTER 1

LOSING WILLIS

JULY 22, 2015, was my thirty-ninth birthday. I was looking forward to what the day would bring (and I was planning to throw a last-minute party of my own on the weekend), but in my exhausted state, my biggest present would be to sleep in. I'd just worked a string of shifts and was well beyond fatigued. Much to my displeasure, the phone rang a few times. I groaned, rolled over, put my phone on airplane mode, and went back to sleep.

I managed to catch a couple more hours of sleep and finally roused myself to do my morning meditation, a ritual I deeply value before facing the frenzy of the emergency department. Even on days I wasn't scheduled to work, I tried not to skip it. After about thirty minutes, I took the phone off airplane mode and the insistent ringing started immediately.

These calls were so persistent I found myself thinking, "Maybe I misread the schedule and I'm supposed to be at work? Or did I schedule a meeting?" Whatever it was, I couldn't put it off any longer. I needed to see who was calling.

It was Louis—Dr. Louis Rolston-Cregler, an emergency medicine resident who had attended my alma mater, Morehouse College, a few years after me. He'd become a mentee and a good friend since joining our residency program at Kings County. His voice was shaking as he tried to control his emotions.

"Wassup, Louis?"

"You got a minute?"

"Yeah, man, of course."

He drew a deep breath. "You need to come to the hospital right away. Willis was stabbed. He's in critical condition."

What? My mind froze. I couldn't grasp what I was hearing. *Willis stabbed?* Willis Young was not only my mentee but one of KAVI's employees and most importantly a close friend, almost my little brother.

Young (his nickname to all) was what we at KAVI call a hospital responder. It was a role that we had developed to break the cycle of trauma after violence. Hospital responders support survivors of all kinds of violence by mitigating their trauma, keeping conflicts from escalating, and helping survivors through recovery. Their most important role is often just to be there. Hospital responders sit with frantic families, answering questions and providing a listening ear. The role was modeled on the job description of the "violence intervention specialist" from the Youth ALIVE! program in Oakland, California. Youth ALIVE!, originally called Caught in the Cross Fire, was the first hospital-based violence intervention program and was created in the early 1990s.[1] They provided violence intervention and support for Highland Hospital, the major public hospital and trauma center in Oakland. Highland Hospital is similar to both Cook County Hospital and Kings County Hospital. After reading material on their program, we modified it to fit the needs of our team and our partners from our allied associations, Save Our Streets (SOS) and Man Up! Inc.[2] We tailored our focus to reach patients in the hospital, rather than to manage violent conflicts in the community. We later reintroduced the "violence intervention specialist" position to the KAVI team to do more comprehensive follow-up on our patients and clients, going well beyond their hospitalization.

Willis's goal was to serve as an advocate for patients injured due to intentional violence and to provide support for their families. Part of that support consisted of talking to the patients and their families about how they were feeling and what they were experiencing. A lot of times people just need to articulate their feelings and emotions, not necessarily receive counseling. Willis had been trained—in large part by shadowing hospital staff, including the emergency docs and social workers—to take histories, listen to stories, offer support, and actively intervene when patients showed any hint of seeking revenge. He trained in violence intervention at conferences around the country and did in-person training at Boston Medical Center with members from the facility's Violence Intervention and Advocacy Program (VIAP).[3] Willis's job was to deescalate conflict, prevent retaliation from occurring after an incident, and help prevent conflict from spreading. Unfortunately, those skills hadn't helped him save himself.

Willis was great at his job. He was from the same neighborhood as some of our patients and had been on the edges of the street life that many of them were a part of. As a teen to a young adult, he'd hustled, finding any way possible to get cash to live on—some methods legal and some illegal. He was a Blood, a member of the Bloods gang. But in joining us at KAVI, he'd decided to take a different path and to try to help others join him on that path. He was what we in the violence intervention community call "a credible messenger"—someone who shared the lived experience of the people he was counseling.

I met Willis in 2011. He'd grown up on the new block I'd just moved to in Bed-Stuy, and although he had moved away from the block, he was there daily, sitting on the stoop hanging out with his friends. They might be drinking and smoking, but he always spoke to me. He was a smart and funny kid, twenty-three years old at the time, and looked like he could be one of my relatives. While I was born in Buffalo, my ancestral family is from the Carolinas and so was his. He looked like some of my cousins and we quickly developed a big brother, little brother relationship. Even before formally joining KAVI, he expressed so much interest in what we were doing. He once told me that he thought about being a minister, that he really wanted to help people, but he wasn't ready to get out of the streets yet. "I'll be there soon," he would say. As with many people in their early twenties, he had a lot to learn about managing adult life—like cooking and keeping track of his money. I helped teach him how to prepare meals on a budget, how to manage his finances, how to behave at a business meeting. I remember when he received his first paycheck; it was in a lump sum for three or four months of work. A few days later he showed up at my house on New Year's Eve, loaded down with shopping bags and gifts, wearing a leather sweat suit and a gold-plated chain. He was proud of his new outfit and gifts to give, and I laughed because he laughed telling me his chain wasn't real. I then pulled him to the side to ask if he spent his entire paycheck. He spent most of it but had enough for his rent that month. Without wanting him to feel ashamed, I suggested that he save a percentage of his money in the future because he wasn't always going to get that amount every pay period. I passed on life skills that had been passed to me—we went shopping, got him some pots and pans and groceries. I taught him how to make quick meals and stuff. He was my little brother. How could he be a victim of the violence he worked so hard to prevent?

As a doctor, I was used to giving people the worst imaginable news. I had treated patients with violent injuries for more than ten years in emergency departments in Chicago and now in Brooklyn. I had seen a lot of death, a lot of sorrow, and I had become skilled at keeping a composed demeanor in the face of immense grief. But now the grief was mine; the devastation had happened to someone dear to me and I was living in a nightmare.

To cope and function, I compartmentalized my emotions, something I did when stressed while working in the emergency department, and drove myself to the hospital to check on Willis. It didn't take long to get hyper-focused, shutting out any distracting feelings or intense emotions so I could get to the hospital safely. I knew emotions were a part of life, but I couldn't afford to be distracted by or lost in them. It was somewhat of a hardened way of dealing with problems but it was how I managed them. In the emergency department you really can't get distracted by peripheral matters when it's busy and patients have life-threatening problems, because they are depending on you to keep them alive.

As I approached Kings County Hospital, I kept up a running

monologue in my head: "Young's tough as shit. He's gonna be al-right. He'll go to the OR, have that surgery, and it'll just take a few weeks for him to get back to working out. He'll be back ringing my doorbell to go running or hit the gym. He'll be back to doing muscle-ups on the pull-up bar in the park and eating the food in my kitchen before asking me in no time."

As I pulled up to the hospital, the running commentary in my mind took a turn: "What happened? This is fucked up, this is so fucked up." Every time Young did something he referred to as grimy or uncouth, something he knew I'd consider dumb or out of character, he'd tell our friends, "Don't let the doc know." That was his respectful but gently mocking name for me. Did he get caught up in some shit he didn't want "the doc" to know about? Maybe, but none of that mattered now.

Willis would never specifically say what he was caught up in, but I assumed it was illegal. I knew that he was struggling every day and I knew that for someone in Willis's position, that some-times meant hustling on the other side of the law. Whenever I asked about it, he would tell me not to worry, that he would be OK. He always said, "I can't get you involved in my shit." I'd al-ways tell him, "Don't do anything stupid that's gonna get you in trouble, arrested, or killed." He replied, "I get it, I get it" with his head hanging down.

Even with whatever he was doing on the side, he often struggled to find necessities like food and shelter. He lost his first apartment after a rent hike; after that, he slept in random places, my couch included. After a while, he found a room on Atlantic Avenue. It was small but it was his and he could lock the door. He appreciated that, but in reality, it was no kind of place to live—an illegally rented storage room in a warehouse. It had no bathroom or kitchen. He had a sleeping bag, some books, and a few plastic urinals. He showered at the nearby gym he went to. It hurt my heart that I couldn't do more. I gave him a little bit of money sometimes or bought groceries or takeout when he was really up against it. I wanted to raise his salary, but we hadn't gotten the funding to do it. He was trying so hard to change his life, but so many cards were stacked against him.

———————

When I arrived at Kings County, I was greeted at the SICU (surgical intensive care unit) by some of my residents. When I looked through the glass doors at the entrance of his room, I saw my friend lying there with bandages over his eye, flank, and abdomen, covering his injuries and post-operative surgical wounds, intubated, on a ventilator, attached to a monitor, with different IV fluids, antibiotics, and blood, running into his veins. It was one of the most brutal stabbings I'd ever seen. The only reason he hadn't died immediately was that he was so young and strong. I thought—I hoped—that that would carry him through.

How could this have happened?

Who did this?

What was he involved in?

Had he been fighting back, trying to defend himself?

The questions ran through my mind over and over, but there were no answers.

I'm someone who has to keep moving. In a crisis, using my body helps me keep my mind right. I used to run competitively. I've given that up, but I snowboard, I train in Brazilian jiu-jitsu, I skateboard. Sometime during that horrible day, I thought, *I've got to get out of here.*

I had been talking to so many people around the hospital, piecing together the story, but it was still all a jumble. I had my skateboard in my trunk and I felt—I knew—that I needed to be alone with my thoughts. I had to figure out what's going to happen next and what we need to do. We needed to raise money. What happens now? I just rode my skateboard around Flatbush. I had my headphones. I skated around thinking, "Alright, he's still alive." After a while, I felt able to go back in and be present. I stayed all day. I didn't have a shift that day, but I had shifts later that week. I would check on him any minute I could.

Willis was in the SICU for two more weeks. More surgeries and more blood transfusions. He still had a lot of life in him and whenever his sedation wore off he "bucked the vent," and tried to pull out the endotracheal tube from his mouth, which was connected to the ventilator breathing for him. Being awake on a ventilator was uncomfortable and had been described by people as waking up with the sensation of a big straw in the back of the throat. One day, I was able to steal away from my shift in the emergency department and visit him briefly. He squeezed my hand and I had a flash of hope. He even opened his uncovered eye. I thought, "Yeah, he's gonna be good. He'll come back like the Bionic Man or the Terminator or something."

So many of his friends and family came to visit him every day, even some of the emergency department staff. Young had touched a lot of lives and we were all hoping for a miracle. My many years of practice in masking my emotions when I talked to families who were coping with death or gravely injured loved ones did me no good. I couldn't hide from my despair as Young's condition took one step forward, two steps back. The two weeks passed in a brokenhearted fog. I kept working but was increasingly distracted and keeping myself isolated.

Then there was the day I was on my way to move my car because of New York's unique (and annoying) alternate-side-of-the-street parking rules. I had just parked when Ty, my neighbor, caught my eye. Our usual "wassup" and throwing the peace sign was forgotten.

"Tell me he didn't die." Ty said, his voice shaking.

What the fuck, I silently said to myself. This had to be street hearsay, where someone misinterpreted the information and didn't realize that critical condition didn't mean death. Yeah, that was it. He couldn't be dead. My body knew the truth while my mind still denied it. Almost immediately, I called Young's uncle, still trying to convince myself that things were alright.

All he could do was confirm the truth of Ty's words. Willis had died at seven that morning, at the age of twenty-seven, another in the long, long list of Black men lost to violence in America.

Weeks later, I learned the answers to some of my questions about how Young had ended up in the SICU. The circumstances tell of a heartbreaking cycle. Young was out at a bar with some guys he knew, one of them named Chad Hollingsworth. After a night of drinking, witnesses said, there was an argument between the two over a woman. I don't know what was said and don't really care, but whatever it was, it led Hollingsworth to savagely attack Young. There was no de-escalation of the incident mentioned. No mention of anyone talking about calming down, being the bigger person, or just walking away. I'm sure there were witnesses to the scuffle—but there was no word of anyone willing to intervene, to break up the fight, to talk them off the ledge. And at least one of them was armed with a knife. Two young Black men, full of potential. And after this encounter one was dead at the hands of the other. In 2017, Hollingsworth received a sentence of three to ten years in prison. Who knows what the rest of his life will be like when he gets out? He might even be out now, but I haven't heard his name mentioned since the conviction.

I don't know all of the circumstances that took place the night Willis was stabbed, and I never will. What I do know is that two lives were lost. Willis was killed and Chad imprisoned. Both of their families lost loved ones. I still mourn the loss of Willis and think about him often (I've yet to delete his cell phone number). But Chad's conviction didn't ease my mind. Another Black man imprisoned didn't make me feel any happier. What does justice being served actually mean? The problem wasn't fixed; it just shifted. I've never known prison to be rehabilitative for anyone, and when Chad was released, what was next?

There are those who find their way inside of prison and develop the skills to become community leaders. Some of our staff at KAVI have been incarcerated in the past and have made their way to just that. But the odds are against them. All of them, if they could turn back time, would do everything possible to avoid prison and the situations that landed them there. Chad may end up as just another Black man destroyed by the system.

In an ideal situation, Willis and Chad would have had the skills to calm down that night, or others around them would have calmed them. The next day, they could have had a conversation with a mediator from the community and aired out their grievances. They would have opened up about the conflict, acknowledging that feelings were hurt, and they would have determined what their common core values were, established a shared ground, reestablished trust, and identified things that could be triggering in the future. They could have come up with a plan, short-term and long-term, that would have ensured this conflict would be resolved and that would have lowered the odds of it flaring up again. That scenario is what we work toward every day at KAVI.

I was in disbelief at the news of Young's passing because I had just seen him the day before and he had squeezed my hand, but I knew the scenario all too well and trying to conjure up ways to avoid the reality of harsh news was common when people learned of an untimely death. Begrudgingly, I walked up the stairs of my building. It was the slowest and most painful walk I'd taken, but at the same time I wanted to hurry and get inside the apartment to be alone as soon as possible to mourn my fallen friend. I collapsed in the doorway of my apartment and stayed there for an hour or more crying.

My tears were for my friend, but they were also for the ongoing cycle that hurts and kills so many, a cycle that will only be broken when we change our approach, as a country, to managing violence and trauma as a public health issue, not as a carceral one. I had formed KAVI out of this conviction and Young had worked every day by my side to help make this change a reality. In his name, in the name of all those who have suffered and died, I want to keep moving forward. We must keep moving forward. But before we can do that, I need to look back. Look back at where I come from. I could have easily been the one lying in that SICU. I know the outcomes of the streets very well. I was lucky—I regularly had extensive support that many in the community didn't have. But I'd seen what can happen. I know it could have happened to me.

CHAPTER 2

JUMPED

IN 1988, I was eleven years old, a sixth grader at Philippa Schuyler Middle School for the Gifted and Talented in the Black and Latino Bushwick neighborhood of Brooklyn, long before it became the gentrified neighborhood it is now. Back then, it was still dotted with the remains of the industrial area it had once been, mixed with a multitude of discount stores, houses with aluminum siding, and bodegas. Schuyler was a haven where the teachers expected students to work hard and excel in academics; we also expected it from each other. I weighed no more than ninety pounds, a nerdy kid who loved *Star Wars*, GI Joe, and comic books.

My route coming home from school was uncomplicated. I got out of school and took the B54 bus down Myrtle Avenue to Carlton Avenue in Fort Greene, just a few miles from Schuyler. It was less than a two-minute walk home from the bus stop, unless I went first into the bodega to get some candy and a "quarter water," a highly sugared drink with food coloring that cost twenty-five cents. Usually, that might be all the excitement I would have before watching my afternoon cartoons and *Video Music Box*, the first Black music video show in the country. But this day was different. This day, shortly after I got off the bus, I got jumped. Two guys who were probably just a little bit older than me—but a lot bigger—grabbed me from behind, punched me in the face and stomach, causing me to double over, and then dug in my pockets. All I had on me was a dollar, my saxophone mouthpiece, and the city-issued bus pass that I used to go to school—slim pickings. They ran off after my neighbor Cinque yelled and chased them away. Cinque, then in his early twenties, lived with his father, Bill Lee, and his stepmother and siblings just two doors down from us. Cinque's older brother was this young Black filmmaker named Spike Lee, whose first film, *She's Gotta Have It*, came out a year and a half before. At the time of this incident, Spike was grown and gone, well on the way to his worldwide success as a filmmaker—I met him but didn't know him. Our families were close: I used to sit on their stoop daily playing with their family dog, Baron, a small brown dachshund. Mr. Lee was also my first music teacher and taught all the kids on the block how to sing and about harmonies and musical scales.

For all the toughness of Fort Greene at this time, it was a community where people looked out for each other and took care of each other. We lived on the third floor in a railroad-style apartment of a four-story walk-up brownstone. I didn't think about whether we lived in a middle-class or in an impoverished neighborhood because I didn't have that vocabulary. It was home. Walt Whitman public housing, where most of the residents were at or close to poverty level, was less than three hundred feet from the door to our apartment. I had friends who lived there—and in the Ingersoll Houses across the street from Whitman—who I played with and visited regularly like Alvin and Israel (Izzy), and I also played with the kids on Myrtle Ave around the corner like Bruce and Alex, Janean, Charmaine, Zach and Charlette, and the kids on my street like Chad, Rahsaan, Malik, Kyiesha, Squeeze, and Peter. Sometimes a few of us would play in our apartment and sometimes I would go over to theirs, and when it started getting late we went home. I wasn't discouraged from playing with the kids around the neighborhood, so I never thought about class. We had a sprinkling of white people on the block, and some Latinos, but the neighborhood was predominantly Black folks. There were schoolteachers, office managers, construction workers, artists, filmmakers, and musicians who lived on the block. Until I got much older I didn't realize how multidimensional and multifaceted our neighborhood was. I'm grateful that I grew up there.

But that edge existed too. And being jumped was still being jumped. Cinque comforted me as he walked me back to my building. I was still shaking and crying but I didn't ask him to come in with me. I was trying to be OK on my own. I wasn't dead, and was physically fine, aside from some minor bumps, but definitely afraid.

My parents weren't home from work yet and I let myself in, still crying but trying to hold it together so I didn't feel like a pussy, but also trying to decide if I was going to tell them. Moms would be home in thirty minutes to an hour. That didn't give me long to think. I was trying to figure out if I could pull myself together enough to avoid telling the whole story or at least minimize the details of what happened. Or maybe I could just not tell them and come up with a different way to get to school. It was a few miles away though so I'd have to leave much earlier than usual, which would arouse suspicion, so that wouldn't work. But if I could figure out how to get out of the house, I could sneak on the back of the bus when it was crowded. I wouldn't have been alone because kids always bum-rushed the back of the bus and the bus driver didn't even blink or seem to care because it would take too long to check to see if we all had our bus passes. But—wait, no—the bus wasn't crowded enough in the morning for that to work, so I would have to pay. My allowance wouldn't cover the bus fare to school for a week. I would need money to get on the bus to get to school now that I didn't have a bus pass. And I did want to keep riding the city bus. I definitely didn't want the fate of those kids who rode the dreaded "cheese bus" (that's what we called traditional yellow school buses). My friends and I laughed at kids who took those or who arrived in private van or car services to middle school. In our minds it was so elementary school, just for little kids—even though I had been in elementary school less than two years before. And anyway, when I thought about it more, I realized that when Cinque inevitably saw my folks on the block, he would tell them what had happened. There was no way out. I had to tell them myself.

My folks were aware of the violence that was out there in the neighborhood and in the city. We had conversations about being aware of my environment and not talking to strangers. Even with all the conversations, I never thought something would happen so quickly on my way home. I also thought that I was the least likely person to be robbed since I had nothing worth stealing except my student bus pass, which offered unlimited rides until about 7 p.m. Monday to Friday. That could add up if the thief wanted to get around for a while.

I was still crying when my mother got home, but I eventually got out the story so that she could understand. She comforted me but didn't freak out, at least not outwardly. She asked if I was OK and let me talk and vent. My father was the same; he just asked if I felt ready to go back to school the next day. I said I was, but in fact I felt violated and vulnerable. More importantly, I wondered, would it happen again?

My parents were, and are, role models of activism and service. My mother, Pat Curry, was an elementary school teacher in neighboring Bed-Stuy. She loved working with what she teasingly called "knucklehead students." It was more of a nickname than a negative label. To her, knuckleheads were those who followed their own path. They were all highly intelligent but were sometimes age-appropriately goofy or what some perceived as disruptive. A lot of teachers who weren't comfortable teaching Black or Brown boys would label them problem kids, treating them like they were much older than they were and punishing them for acting their actual ages. The students who were often sent to her class had many times been labeled "unteachable" and "slow." As the mother of a Black boy and the educator of Black and Brown kids, she took the work personally and made it her mission to help them become the best possible students they could become.

My father, Bob Gore ("Pop" as I call him), brought his activism both to his job in the television industry and to his passion, photography. As a young man, he was a community organizer in the Southern Christian Leadership Conference (SCLC), one of the primary organizations leading the fight for civil rights in the 1960s.

Later, as deputy director of WNYC, one of New York City's public broadcasting organizations, he helped create the only prime-time, regularly scheduled Black programming in the country. He was the New York State campaign manager for Jesse Jackson when Jackson ran for president in 1984. On the side my father was a photographer for many prominent African American institutions, among them the Schomburg Center for Research in Black Culture, Pathways to College, the Congressional Black Caucus, and the New York NAACP. He saw his professional and volunteer work as an extension of the civil rights work of his youth. I was lucky to have them both—supportive, loving parents who were always there for me.

Not everyone had that. Even before I got jumped, I knew that the world outside was often a far different beast than the safe haven I enjoyed at school or at home with my parents. Not long after I got jumped, a couple of months later, while at home, I heard a loud pop-pop! I looked out the window to see what the noise was, hoping they were firecrackers, which I loved. People played with firecrackers all summer long on the block and in the park. But as the sound continued, I realized that it didn't sound like regular firecrackers exploding. That's when I saw the two guys running down the street with black guns. I'd heard gunshots before on a shooting range and off in the distance at night, but these were different and seemed more real because they were less than fifty feet away. I got scared and immediately ducked down and ran away from the window. I don't remember anyone formally telling me to duck if you hear gunshots, maybe I got it from war movies on TV, maybe I just had that instinctive reaction. Eventually the shots stopped and the regular sounds of the neighborhood— voices, horns, radios, and revving car and bus engines—seemed to take over the soundscape again. This was the height of the crack era, and the drug was spreading like a murderous wildfire. The pop-pop-pop sounds echoed outside would become more frequent, telling of the danger they brought. Daily life went on, but alongside it there were violent scenes, like the one I saw, and sad scenes of people jittering on the street corners, "fiending for a hit." My friends and I were always leery of "crackheads." You didn't want one of them running up on you to rob you, and it was creepy to see a person who became a zombie shaking near you. It was almost as if I might get what they had if they touched me. As they became more and more prevalent on the streets, I learned to constantly scan my surroundings—practically everyone was a perceived threat.

In the 1980s, in Fort Greene as well as Bushwick, the neighborhood my school was in, all of us got robbed at some point. We all made defensive moves like putting our dollars in our socks and changing up the routes we took to school and staying partnered up. In some ways, it was kind of a unifying factor. But that didn't make it any easier.

After I got jumped, fear followed me every time I walked out the door of our apartment. I wasn't fidgety. I didn't have signs of anxiety, like having a hard time breathing when going into unfamiliar places. But I did become extra analytical—hyperaware and more cautious of people and the environment. Maybe it was innocence lost or a new awareness of how some people could treat others. I didn't become depressed or isolate myself, but my hyperawareness of the community and details of my surroundings became a reflex. Now it's something I see often in people I treat, albeit at a heightened level. Not wanting to feel like a victim, I asked my mother if I could take karate lessons to give me some sense that I could protect myself. I also changed up the route going to school and coming home, opting for a busier street with regular foot traffic and a better reputation. In the sneaker culture that pervaded the neighborhood at the time, I knew that nobody would steal my beat-up sneakers—my parents got them straight from the ten-dollar discount bin at Modell's, much to my frustration, but at least I could hide money in them.

My parents knew about and approved of the route change and said I could take karate. What they didn't know was that I started carrying razor blades, box cutters, screwdrivers, or anything else I could think of to strike back. I'd used box cutters often when I worked with my father, opening boxes, cutting matting for pictures, or cutting the edges of things neatly, their intended purpose. I'd seen older guys tuck rectangular razor blades inside their cheek, and with a flick of the tongue they'd hold it between their teeth, ready to use in an attack. But the notion of it as a weapon for me to use was new. It was magical thinking, a totem of protection. I knew it could be used as a weapon and that a person could get badly sliced up with it, but I'd never thought about how I would even pull it out to use it when I needed it. I never practiced with it, and given that I was a thin eleven-year-old—not a movie superhero or a ninja—it was highly unlikely I would have successfully defended myself even if I had. The razor blades were props in my pocket to give me confidence. Maybe I thought instinct would naturally set in if I got jumped. *I'll be ready next time*, I'd mutter to myself, mustering courage from somewhere in my ninety-pound frame. I wasn't a violent kid. I liked to play-fight and wrestle with my friends and cousin, but I'd much rather read comic books and watch *Star Wars*. I wanted to feel safe. I needed some sense of certainty when I walked outside every morning. The instinct to survive made me more acutely aware of my environment because of my trauma. I began studying people's facial expressions as they walked nearby, looking at how they carried themselves, how they navigated the street. Did their walk look hurried, or was there a natural, slow pace? Did the person look anxious, like they were about to do something dangerous? Did they fidget with their hands in their pockets, as though they had a weapon? Or were they just fidgeting because they had loose change in their pockets?

Your perspective changes when the trauma, even if it's not life-threatening, becomes personal. I didn't want to cause anyone any harm. I just wanted to survive.

I was already exhibiting signs of a reaction to trauma, the same kind of trauma that haunts so many others. I had a good support system in my parents and a close community. I had friends and was in a safe and supportive school; there was plenty of heat in our apartment in the colder months and plenty to eat. And even with all that, my ongoing reaction to being jumped was to go into—and stay in—fight mode.

When under threat, humans are hardwired to go into the "defense cascade."[1] *Arousal* is the first step in the cascade: the quickening of my heartbeat and sudden cold sweat and tensing of my muscles that came when the guys grabbed me. The next steps are either *fight* or *flight*, the response to the new threat to my safety. But my perpetrators punched me too quickly and restrained me too effectively for me to respond in either fashion, especially since it was two against one and I was much smaller. Had I anticipated or received the slightest warning, I would have felt a surge of adrenaline that pushed me to fight back or run as fast as I could to get away. Since I couldn't escape, what followed was *immobility* as they punched me. My shaking and crying as they ran off was part of that state. And after that, my hypervigilance and decision to carry weapons with some notion that I could fight back was the deeply rooted remains of that attack. I carry some of that trauma within me still—and my story isn't even close to what I see every day at work, what some people go through every day.

When I think of my eleven-year-old self, packing a box cutter, thinking he could defend himself, I feel sad. Not just because of the disaster that would have ensued had I ever really tried to use that weapon—I was far from causing harm (which I didn't want to do). I most likely would have gotten my own throat cut. But what does it do to a kid to begin to have to make this kind of calculus? It goes beyond robbing them of innocence—it affects the formation of their brains and has a significant effect on the rest of their lives. There is the need to feel powerful and resilient because they've been violated. For some, it becomes a mission to never feel vulnerable again, building a shell around themselves even if that means closing themselves off from the outside world. Even more extreme, the person attacked can vow that it will never happen again and instead of wanting to protect themselves, they turn to become the aggressor, seeking opportunities to establish a tough persona, seeking to become the predator instead of the prey. This happens regularly to young and even older people, who I could tell were genuinely pleasant and friendly but have been so hardened by repeated traumas that they are now shells of their former selves, unable to live without fear and insecurity. They're closed off from the outside world because of the fear that something bad will come about from engaging in a new or different experience.

The social support systems we have within our communities have the ability to provide informational, emotional, physical, and even financial aid.[2] They can help build additional safety nets after a person has experienced trauma, which help create a level of balance and getting the individual back to normal living as much as is possible. The goal of the support systems, counseling and therapy included, should not be to help the traumatized individual forget the experience but to have a more in-depth awareness, to help them work through challenges and adapt to a way of living after going through the trauma. In the aftermath of something horrendous, we would love to never have to think about it, be triggered to relive it, but forgetting doesn't really happen; the emotions just get tucked away, growing, festering, and eventually emerging with new stressors or triggers. Pretending otherwise is damaging. The trauma needs to be confronted and worked through.

Support can exist in many places. It can be found in family, a church or mosque or temple, school, an after-school program, or from a guidance counselor. At KAVI, not only do we provide immediate support to those seeking help, but we guide them to further mental health support in the wake of their trauma. Talking to friends is one thing but sometimes the voice of someone with specialized training and expertise is what's needed. Support needs to come from every direction.

From the perspective of years later, I know that those kids who jumped me just wanted to survive too. The minuscule amount of money stolen could have been used to buy food or snacks. The punches I received may have been a way for them to practice becoming a predator to be feared, not prey. The tools they used weren't healthy ones from my perspective of being on the receiving end of the blows, but for the kids in my neighborhood growing up, who had no resources to help them think of any other way to live, that behavior was acceptable. I don't know what happened to those kids. I didn't see them again or at least didn't recognize them; nor do I know what their home lives were like. But there's a strong possibility that a number of them had grown up around what are known as adverse childhood experiences (ACEs).

In the late 1980s and 1990s, Dr. Vincent Felitti, a preventive med-icine specialist in California, was looking to figure out why more than half of the patients enrolled in his successful obesity clinic dropped out. While interviewing some of those patients, there was a noticeable pattern: more than two hundred of the obese patients had been sexually abused. His team began to realize that many of the patients they saw with unmanaged obesity had suffered one or more traumatic experiences in their childhood. Intrigued by this, Dr. Felitti, Dr. Robert Anda, and other researchers designed an in-depth study to look at correlations between ACEs and health conditions in adults. Their "ACE Study" was conducted with the private healthcare giant Kaiser Permanente and the government's Centers for Disease Control with 17,421 patients enrolled; the results were published in 1998 under the title "The Relation Be-tween Adverse Childhood Experiences and Adult Health."[3] In the study, patients were asked ten questions exploring their upbring-ing. They were asked specifically about

Physical abuse (hitting, punching, kicking, etc.) by someone in the household
Sexual abuse (sexual assault, rape, sexual exploitation of a
child)
Emotional abuse (such as threatening, isolating, blam-
ing, etc.)
Physical neglect (not providing adequately for basic needs
of food and shelter)
Emotional neglect (failing to provide social support or
needed mental health treatment, also not responding to
a child's entreaties—ignoring pleas for food or warmth,
for example)
Mental illness in a household member
Living with a formerly incarcerated person
Witnessing violence against the mother or other family
members
Alcohol or substance abuse in the home

> Parental divorce or separation (if there is great animosity, custody fights, etc.)

In the opening paragraphs of the report, the doctors wrote:

A striking finding was that adverse childhood experiences are vastly more common than recognized or acknowledged. Of equal importance was our observation that they had a powerful correlation to adult health a half-century later. It is this combination that makes them so important. Slightly more than half of our middle-class population of Health Plan members experienced one or more of the categories we studied. One in four was exposed to two categories of abusive experience, one in 16 to four categories. Given an exposure to one category, there is 80% likelihood of exposure to another. All this, of course, is well shielded by social taboos against obtaining this information. Further, one may "miss the forest for the trees" if one studies these issues individually. They do not occur in isolation; for instance, a child does not grow up with an alcoholic person or with domestic violence in an otherwise well-functioning household. The question to ask is: How will these childhood experiences play out decades later in a doctor's office? How does one perform reverse alchemy, going from a normal newborn with almost unlimited potential to a diseased, depressed adult? How does one turn gold into lead?

To put it more bluntly and briefly, people who have a lot of bad shit happen to them growing up have trouble maintaining healthy habits and generally don't live as long as those who escaped that. The scary fact is that more than 60 percent of the US population has at least one ACE.[4] According to the Compassion Prison Project, 97 percent of those incarcerated have experienced one or more ACE.[5] A study from Wales showed that 84 percent of adult male prisoners had at least one or more ACE and 45 percent had four or more ACEs.[6] Further, people with one or several ACEs have more propensity toward violence and drug use, often starting in adolescence.[7]

These sad numbers aren't just stats to me; nor are they distant. They are reflected and multiplied with the Black, Brown, immigrant, poor, and working-class patients I care for. My foster brother Angel, who came to us when he was eight and I was eleven, had at least five ACEs. The love and support that my family gave him, while real, wasn't enough. Before I lost Willis, I lost another brother—not to death, but to the streets.

Angel entered the foster care system after one of his sisters was injured by a glass object in their apartment. The kids ended up in the emergency department to be treated, but the injury, though minor, nonetheless triggered a Child Protective Services evaluation. That revealed the significant problems in Angel's home: his mother was hooked on stimulant drugs and pills, and he and his younger sisters were pretty much raising themselves. In an ideal world, they would have gone to live with his grandmother in her apartment to help maintain familial ties and be in a familiar environment, but she had no more space. Her apartment was beyond crowded as some of her own children lived there and she was raising a few of Angel's cousins and his oldest siblings. Angel's father was unable to help because he was in prison. My parents had been open to fostering for years, and when they were contacted, they quickly agreed to bring Angel into our home.

Angel was funny and smart and full of potential—a gifted artist and a thinker. But at age eight his unstable home life had already marked him deeply. He had his quiet moments, but they could turn quickly and he'd get angry and out of control. Angel attended the same school where my mother taught over in Bed-Stuy, so when he acted out, her colleagues came to her with reports of his behavior. He rode with her to school in the morning and home again in the afternoon. She was engaging with him and his challenging behavior from the time she got up until the time she went to bed, caught in the crossfire everywhere she went. And he wasn't her only child of course. I didn't have the same social and behavioral challenges as Angel, but I had a lot of energy that needed to be managed and addressed. My father was home late evenings and the weekends unless he was traveling for work, but my mother bore the brunt of the childcare. She loved Angel and wanted the best for him, but she got burned out. My father also did his best as Angel's only father figure, but he too could only do so much.

Even with all the conflicts Angel had in his life before we met, he and I became close. I had always wanted a brother, so it didn't take much time for me and Angel to bond. Maybe he felt safe with our family. We fought a lot and played a lot, practicing moves we learned from "karate movies," which is what we called any film with martial arts. The "foster" title implied a temporary situation, but as far as I was concerned once the brother bond was formed, it was permanent. I vowed to look out for him, to make sure he was protected and safe, for as long as I could.

I kept that part of the bargain when we were kids. I made sure that people didn't pick on him too much, and I protected him. As he got older, Angel liked to fight more and was good at it. He did the same for me, making sure that no one messed with me. But then things changed.

I had seen the dangers ahead when he was still living with us, including his outbursts of anger that could erupt out of nowhere or with just mild triggers, like someone looking at him. I saw how he seemed to be transported into another realm when he fought, not fully aware of his anger and rage. Some days were better than others, but I couldn't always anticipate what could trigger him. I know now that a lot of his anger stemmed from being away from his family. Despite the family challenges that had landed him in foster care, he also wanted and needed to stay in touch with his biological family. Sometimes I accompanied him to his grandmother's house (his grandmother had continued playing host to a rotating cast of her adult children and their children) over in neighboring Bed-Stuy so he could visit with her. The family was always friendly to me and welcoming, but it was always jarring for me to see how they lived and the poverty Angel had been born into. When I walked into the apartment building, there was graffiti donning the walls and an overwhelming smell of old and new piss.

Graffiti and the smell of piss were nothing new to me. In the 1980s, it was all over New York City—on the trains, parking lots, alleys, and even some apartment buildings. I'd been in public housing plenty of times before. But my friends who lived there had stable home lives—enough to eat, parental and family support, some semblance of order in their lives. When I went into Angel's house with him, it was the first time I'd been in a home where everyone there was just lying around watching TV. The apartment was dirty. Stuff was all over the place. The kids were dirty. None of the adults had jobs, or even side hustles—working at a store or maybe doing construction on the sly. I remember seeing roaches running around on the counter. Everyone I knew in Brooklyn had roaches on occasion. But I'd never seen them crawling out of multiple cereal boxes and bowls onto the counter. It was a big apartment—three or four bedrooms, with the area and space of a house. But there were easily ten people living there. Angel didn't even have a bed to himself.

And yet, even amid that chaos, whenever we left, he'd hug his sisters, brother, cousins, and all of his relatives as if it were the last time he'd see them. There was a beautiful love and family connection, but the family didn't have any of the support or skills needed to thrive. He was torn—he longed for them, but when he was in the quiet, clean stable environment of our apartment, I could tell that he reached a different kind of peace, even when he was acting his toughest.

After a little over two years, his mother successfully completed her court-mandated rehab program and Angel and his sisters were reunited with her (his elder siblings remained at the family's apartment being cared for by other relatives after their grandmother died). Despite our intentions to stay in touch, our weekend visits became monthly and the monthly visits became quarterly. Our conversations changed too. He seemed more and more focused on just surviving, even though he was only in middle school. To make money, he bagged groceries at the supermarket around the corner from where he lived, and he tried to move forward. But life was still highly unstable. At one point he was the only one in the apartment with a job, making him the easy go-to for his mother and other adult relatives to borrow money from. Not the burden to be expected of a kid in middle school.

Later, when I was finishing high school and filling out college applications, Angel started getting involved in the drug game. I'd found out about him being a lookout for drug dealers in "The Stuy" (pronounced *Sty*) and, like a good big brother, I told him to watch out and "stop doing that shit." Lookout kids died just as easily as the dealers, and users had a relatively short life expectancy, we both knew. It wasn't long before he moved up to selling drugs himself.

He'd eventually go to juvie at Spofford while I was away at college, but juvie was just the beginning. When he got out, I was away and didn't see him. We spoke, but only short phone conversations about staying off the streets. He "yessed" me a lot, but I could never tell if my words were effective or fell on deaf ears. Our lives were becoming very different and far more distant. I would move to Atlanta to go to Morehouse College, and he would spend more time in the streets surviving. I don't think I really internalized how difficult it was for him to simply survive, or anyone who has lived in poverty, to fend for themselves. I'd always felt supported and had all the things I needed to be able to live comfortably. My parents never borrowed money from me. My parents were loud talkers, but our apartment was relaxing and peaceful. I'd never had to share my bed or personal space with anyone other than visiting relatives. No one in my immediate family had gone to prison yet. It was almost like I lived in an ivory tower of support. I *did* live in an ivory tower of support.

Ultimately, Angel succumbed fully to the allure of the street. While I was at Morehouse, he would be convicted of armed robbery. Even though he was seventeen, still a minor, he was sentenced as an adult and sent off to prison.

I was getting more and more caught up in my own life. When I came home for semester break, I never went up to visit him upstate and I felt really shitty about it. Even worse, I only wrote him one letter the entire time I was in college. He called infrequently, always collect, as prisoners were required to. There was always so much pain in his voice that it was hard for me to know what to say. I didn't know if I should try to joke with him or be serious, so the conversations felt awkward and extra short. I thought about him a lot but couldn't fathom what he was going through. I felt guilty for being free and thought I had failed him by not being empathetic or even available. I knew it wasn't my burden to bear at the age of twenty, but perhaps because I was twenty I also felt like it was my fault he had gotten so lost. When we were both adults, more than twenty years later, Angel disclosed to me that his mother went back to using drugs not long after the family was reunited. He would frequently be hungry and his only focus was survival. He had to be able to take care of himself by any means, and if it couldn't be done legally, making money illegally would at least keep him fed and clothed.

Ultimately, he ended up at a detention center in Brooklyn. It was still a lockdown situation, but it was closer to home, another step closer to freedom. While home on summer break, I decided to see him. I was nervous about being searched and questioned in order to get in, but I was much more worried about how prison might have changed Angel. Going in was just as bad as I'd feared. I remember metal tables, heavy metal doors, being buzzed in, and getting checked and frisked by officers. I remember everything was plain and drab, almost lifeless. There was nothing vibrant or welcoming. I was so conflicted: I wanted to see him and make sure he was OK, but I also wanted to get the hell out of there. Once I got through and into the visiting area, there he was. My brother, smiling but sad. He apologized to me for having to see him locked up, dressed in prison garb. We cried together a little bit but then pulled ourselves together and joked around and talked about old times. I could tell he didn't want to talk about his time upstate or in the current detention center, so we kept the conversation light. All too soon, visiting time ended. He was taken through another set of security doors, deeper into the heart of the building, and I was led through a set of security doors in the opposite direction. Once he was out of sight, I couldn't hold it together anymore. As soon as I got beyond those heavy metal doors, I sunk into the wall, easing to sit on the floor, and cried. They weren't the joyful tears of reunion but tears of guilt, anger, frustration, and regret. I cried because of the pain of where he was and the guilt of where I was. We were supposed to be successful together. Prison wasn't part of the plan.

We continued to drift apart. I thought about him a lot, and hoped he was safe. I always felt like I could have done more. But I was just a kid myself. I wished I could undo all the ills that he had been through and have him find some semblance of peace in his life. Angel never had the support he so badly needed. My parents did their best but there were limits to what they could provide, particularly once Angel returned to his biological family. His family needed support and guidance themselves, and that should have been part of a humane system, one that gives kids like Angel comprehensive support, that provides basic resources for him and his family, and that supports mental health and addresses deep familial trauma. He'd always been a talented artist and would sit undisturbed for hours and hours drawing, sketching, creating, and coloring his work. Maybe he would have been an artist or game designer, maybe designed clothes, who knows? We'll never know.

My father stayed in contact with Angel. He would get occasional collect calls from whichever prison he was in at the time and would send him whatever care packages were allowed to be sent behind the walls. But I didn't see Angel again until 2017 when he was released from another prison stint. He went back to prison and jail numerous times, getting hooked on stimulant pills while there. We hung out once or twice, but he was always jittery, sweaty, distracted—the telltale signs of withdrawal.

I was on a Saturday morning shift at Brooklyn's Kings County Hospital when Angel was brought in for having suicidal thoughts. We connected briefly, and I regularly checked on him during my shift, but each time I went into his room I realized we were in different universes. In the tumult of the emergency department, and while I was caring for patients, I couldn't spend quality time with him to really connect in the way he deserved. He was evaluated by psychiatry and eventually discharged to his residence. His expression and talk of suicide were deemed a result of intoxication. He stopped talking about suicide once he sobered up but remained tearful and in pain. My hope was that his depression, anxiety, and substance abuse would be managed in outpatient clinics. I don't know if that ever happened. He disappeared and I didn't hear from him for years. I didn't know if he was still alive.

While writing this book, five years later, I received a phone call from a New York City hospital asking if I was Angel's brother. I was hoping this wasn't a phone call for me to identify his body and thankfully it wasn't. Angel was alive but in serious condition. He'd arrived in the hospital's emergency department, in an altered state and confused, with a high fever, the result of sepsis, microorganisms in the blood that can compromise some of the body's organ systems and even cause death. While on high doses of IV antibiotics to treat the infection, Angel's mental status improved and he was able to tell the medical team he had a brother who was a doctor. Skeptical of what he was telling the team, they nevertheless had an eager and helpful medical student named Luke who googled me to see if I was real person. He later contacted my hospital, who then contacted me to alert me of the severity of Angel's medical condition. After more than five years of wondering if Angel was still alive, I would see him face-to-face.

I walked into the hospital, one I'd been to quite a few times before to visit other relatives who were patients or to have meetings with colleagues. I saw him, emaciated, confined to a bed, and a shell of himself. His voice was the same but with an exorbitant amount of pain in it. I was happy that he was alive but scared for how long he would survive. He had been living on the streets since I'd last seen him and got even more heavily into drugs. Alcohol, weed, and crack weren't strong enough to cover the pain he frequently spoke about in his hospital room. He began using opiates, first taking pills but realizing his physical pain could be numbed much more quickly with IV drugs. "I would use more than twenty bags of fentanyl in a few days if I could," he told me. The heavy use of narcotics lowered the threshold of his pain tolerance, requiring him to use opiates almost daily. His intravenous drug use with contaminated needles would eventually lead to bacterial seeding throughout his body, leaving abscesses and collections of pus embedded in muscles throughout his body, requiring multiple surgeries to treat.

He also had osteomyelitis, infections of the bone, requiring regular doses of IV antibiotics. My bright, creative, and formerly energetic brother was now confined to a hospital bed with life-threatening infections. As his brother, I was optimistic that he would heal from his infections and go into rehab, coming out renewed after maybe a year. However, my skeptical medical brain of more than twenty years of practice suggested that the majority of patients afflicted with deep-seated trauma and substance abuse did not fare well without extensive support, wraparound services, and a willing participant. I was hoping the optimistic side of me would triumph along with Angel's health.

I tried not to keep repeating the mantra "If I could go back in time" because it wouldn't fix anything and it made me feel depressed, falling into the realm of "I could have, would have, should have." I could only move forward and be supportive to others to the best of my abilities. Like so many others who work with youth with challenges, I've had to stop internalizing other people's problems and making them my own. But the work I do is to honor all those who've been lost and those who are still struggling to heal.

Angel was a lot like some of the kids and patients who come to us in KAVI—energetic and highly intelligent but severely traumatized as a result of ACEs. We try to ameliorate the damage of this trauma and allow them to move toward their full potential, a chance Angel and Willis never got.

CHAPTER 3

F THE POLICE

IN THE SPRING OF 1991, I was a freshman at Brooklyn's Bishop Loughlin Memorial High School. My day-to-day routine consisted of going to school, studying, chasing after teenage girls, and track practice. Outside of school, however, just as it was for every young Black guy I knew, racial tension was on my mind. In the back of our consciousness was a world in which we weren't safe. Not safe in our own Black and Latino neighborhoods, not safe in the larger white world. Where were we safe? Hard to say. As a young Black man, I lived every day with a fear of not just being harmed but of being killed. The vivid images of violence and blatant racism were haunting but very real and present.

I was particularly attuned to these images from the news and talks with my family. My father was intimately acquainted with the story of fourteen-year-old Emmett Till, a native Chicagoan who had been visiting relatives in the Mississippi Delta area. Till was brutally murdered at the hands of a group of white thugs, some of whom were police, because a white woman, Carolyn Bryant Donham, accused him of whistling at her and making lewd comments. While she claimed that she didn't know what would be done to him because of such an accusation, it's hard to believe that a Southern woman at this time would have no idea of the fate that awaited Emmett. Emmett was beaten to death and thrown into a river where his face and body were mangled from being wound up in a river-boat motor. Till's story hit close to home for my father, as he was also from Chicago and visited family in the Deep South during the summers. Whether a boy whistled at a white woman is a moot point—his crime was being Black. Like America during and prior to the civil rights era, it wasn't much different in 1991. The age-old tradition of discounting and dishonoring Black bodies continued.

My father kept copies of *Ebony* and *Life* magazines of the time showing harrowing pictures of Till's mutilated body in the coffin. He made sure I saw these images and knew the history that surrounded them so that I'd be cautious but also have an even greater understanding and awareness of racism. He made sure I knew of not just the darkness but the heroism of the civil rights movement. The PBS documentary *Eyes on the Prize* was required annual viewing in my home.

The attacks came fast and furious in the late 1980s and early '90s. In 1989, a young Black man, Yusuf Hawkins, was killed by a white kid in the predominantly white neighborhood of Bensonhurst in Brooklyn, a subway ride from Fort Greene. Hawkins had gone there with his cousin to purchase a car. He and a couple of his friends were chased with bats by a mob of about thirty guys. One of them had a gun—he pulled it out and shot Yusuf in the chest.

In March of 1991, another Black man named Rodney King had the shit beat out of him by four cops from the Los Angeles Police Department. King had been driving down I-210 when he was pulled for suspicion of intoxication. Four cops piled on him and beat him unconscious, even though he was offering them no resistance—one of the first racist incidents of this kind to be widely broadcast because it was captured on video. King's battered face reminded me of the images of Till that I'd seen so often. From the video, anyone can see that Mr. King wasn't resisting arrest and that *more* than excessive force was used. My friends and I, the Black guys I knew, all saw it and we all felt "that could have been me. If I'd been in the wrong place at the wrong time, that could have been me."

There were so many images of Black death that it was overwhelming, and they kept coming. Right after the merciless Rodney King beating and also in Los Angeles, a Korean grocery store owner shot and killed a fifteen-year-old Black girl named Latasha Harlins. She was in the ninth grade, the same grade as me. Latasha was accused of stealing a bottle of orange juice and the grocery store owner, shot her in the back of the head. She was found to have two dollars clenched in her fist, likely to be used to purchase the orange juice.

A few weeks before I started school in the fall of 1991, there were riots and protests happening in nearby Crown Heights after a Black Guyanese boy named Gavin Cato was hit by a car driven in an Orthodox Jewish motorcade. The car apparently sped up to beat the traffic light, hit another car, and then swerved and hit Gavin and his cousin while they played in front of their apartment building.[1] There were different versions of the incident, but one that seemed to light the fuse of the brewing tensions between the Black and Jewish communities in Crown Heights was that the Jewish-run ambulance company, Hatzolah, was ordered by the cops to pick up the Jewish driver of the car, but they left Gavin behind at the scene. Gavin later died from his injuries at nearby Kings County Hospital.[2]

Over and over, Black bodies were treated as expendable. Was I expendable? If I could keep to myself, mind my business, and stay out of white neighborhoods, then maybe I could be safe and minimize any potential threat.

I had no call to be in any white neighborhoods anyway, so the threats there, while they made me angry, were not immediately present. But, sadly, just as when I was in middle school, I had to be on the alert in the neighborhoods where I lived, went to school, and played.

I didn't think about death and being safe all the time, though. I thought about school. I thought about track, and I spent a lot of time thinking about girls. So, if an opportunity to meet some new girls and hang out with them and maybe even get some came up, then that's what I focused on. Getting some was more of a spectrum. Sex (I mean, like, all the way) was welcomed, but it had only happened to me once before. If I could make out with a girl, cop a feel or two, I wasn't doing too badly.

It was Halloween and my boy Derick hit me up and said he met some girl and she had a friend, so I should come through to the crib to kick it. We had the day off from school (one of the benefits of going to a Catholic high school was they always let us out for Halloween).

The girls came by the house and I could tell immediately that I was Derick's wingman—this one girl was really into him. But it was cool because her friend was quite friendly. . . . And I got to make out with her, and we all had fun kicking it the rest of the afternoon.

After a couple of hours, it was time to catch the bus home and then kiss and go our separate ways. The light was beginning to escape the sky and shifting the feel of the neighborhood. It was kind of cool looking; you could appreciate the details of the trees and houses, but as night fell, well-lit blocks and corners transformed into dark spaces with shadows where unsuspected things or people could emerge from.

On our way to the bus stop, a group of five to six Black guys wearing hoodies yelled over to us from across the street, "Yo, wassup!" Wassup meant many things. It could be a greeting, a question—or a summons to fight. Neither of us knew any of the guys. As they began crossing the street, Derick calmly shouted, "Wassup" back—and shook a construction-grade metal bolt from his sleeve. He pointed it at the group in self-defense, as a threat. Derick had been in fights before and responded reflexively. Like me with my box cutter a few years earlier, he was primed to try to defend himself, even though it probably wouldn't have ended well. The guys mumbled some obscenities, left us alone, and kept walking in the opposite direction.

We continued to walk to the bus stop, which was a block and a half away. When we were able to see the bus stop, the bus was already there and less than a hundred feet away. We started to jog to catch it, but the girls said they didn't feel like running and the bus pulled off. I was upset for a couple of reasons: it was cold, and the bus on Kings Highway always took a long time to come.

The four of us waited for about fifteen minutes for the bus to come but not surprisingly, it was nowhere to be seen. While we were waiting, in the midst of small talk, a few guys with hoodies approached—they couldn't have been the same guys from earlier because they came from a different direction. But we stood at the bus stop so long I wondered if they just circled back around. Were they the same guys? Did they call somebody? Was this a new threat? Who knows. But they came out of nowhere, wearing rubber Halloween masks and ski masks—and began walking toward us. Four became eight and eight became twelve and in an instant there were about twenty guys coming at us. I whispered to Derick and the girls that we needed to run and get the hell out of there, but he said to relax. "They'll probably leave us alone since we have girls with us." I doubted it, although about ten of them kept walking past us, making me think for a second that they would actually leave us alone. There was no trouble until the guys in the back of their crew lingered near us. One of them commented, "You have some pretty girls with you." Maybe that was his more-subtle way of saying "wassup." The comment was followed by a "Yo, my man, that's a nice jacket," gesturing to me. As he reached to grab my sleeve I pulled my arm back and mumbled something incomprehensible. I was scared shitless.

All I remember was Derick shouting to me, "Rob, look out!" As I turned toward Derick, a fist just missed my temple but struck me hard in the ear, knocking my baseball cap to the ground. "Run!" In less than a second, the mob of guys without visible faces was chasing us into the super busy Kings Highway traffic. The girls just stood there at the bus stop. We yelled for them to come on and run but they just stood there. Were they too scared to move? Did they know the hooded and masked guys? Did they set us up to be robbed? I have no idea. I couldn't even think about that because Derick and I were still running and dodging cars across the four lanes of the busy street. My cross-country and track skills were deployed with even more focus than in an important meet; I had lung capacity and I was running for my life. Even though I didn't have my box cutter, I knew never to go into someone else's neighborhood unless I was wearing sneakers, which were on my feet. If there was an instance that I needed to run for safety, I was ready.

We finished dodging cars and oncoming traffic and slipped into the McDonald's on the other side of the street by Utica and Avenue H. Panicked and breathing heavily, we ducked behind a table to avoid being noticed, while keeping a lookout for the goons. As we huddled there, hearts pounding, eyes scanning, two white male police officers came in.

On TV, the cops were the good guys, usually working for justice (except for those shows and movies about crooked cops). And I *had* had a good experience with a Black woman officer who had known me since I was a kid and was friends with my mother. I went to elementary school with her daughters, so I was comfortable with her and her family. She was the only cop I knew growing up who didn't give me the creeps. But the other cops I could recognize or identify? No. Mostly what I had learned, from both peers and other adults, was that for folks who looked like me, who lived where we lived, not only were cops unlikely to be of help; they might be the ones after you. I wish I believed that that these officers would help us. But I doubted it. I had long known the drill: I made eye contact with them, kept my hands out of my pocket, and didn't make any sudden movements.

Whether walking down the street to the store or going through the train station, especially if I was traveling with at least one other person, I was profiled. Derick and I had been followed by police officers and plainclothes cops in stores before and had squad cars slow down a few feet from us while walking down the street. I'd been handcuffed before for walking through an open gate in the train station—even though I was right behind a white guy who had just done the same thing. My friends and I had been followed by cops while walking down the street. It didn't matter if I played in the school band, ran cross-country, and was on the honor roll. We were considered criminals on sight, so why should this interaction with them be any different?

"What are you doing in here?" one of the officers shouted at us. Based on the tone of his voice and sheer command, I instantly knew we were suspects. "What is that," he asked, pointing at Derick's metal bolt, before snatching it from him.

"Twenty dudes are chasing us," I replied with a shaking voice because my body was trembling.

They laughed and said, "Get out! You probably did something."

"But, but, but," I stuttered.

"I don't care. Get out!"

After being kicked out of the McDonald's, I could see the guys were still waiting for us outside at the corner. Once we got out of the doors we ran as hard as we could for as long as we could. A few of them chased after us but stopped after a while. I knew I could keep that pace up for a while, and seeing Derick right next to me, I knew that he could too. We kept running until it was clear they were no longer a visible threat.

There were a lot of thoughts running in my skull while my feet were running down the streets. Most of my friends had at one point been chased by guys, sucker punched, or jumped. I had. If it hadn't happened to a kid yet, then there was the expectation that it would happen soon. Since there was potential, there was a need to be ready. Getting jumped wasn't even something worth discussing since it was such a common occurrence. Guys would trade stories around the lunchroom table of being chased, getting jumped, being beaten, and then beating someone up in return, or thinking about retaliation. Maybe the lunchtime stories were part of getting ready and having a better understanding of the environment and were an integral and, sadly, necessary part of our rites of passage. For Black boys especially, there's an ethos of being tough, of shaking off these events. I took part in it myself in a small way and I see it writ large with my patients. Even if they are terrified and showing it when they first come in, so often they throw up a screen of bravado the minute they're stabilized. That toughness is one of the community norms that we badly need to break down. The "tough-guy" veneer so many kids of color, especially those growing up in poverty, typically adopt actually works against them, preventing them from admitting their fears and vulnerabilities, from getting the support and protection they badly need.

Being bullied and threatened didn't need to be a rite of passage that we all went through. My jacket wasn't even worth stealing. We had no prior beef with the group of guys. We just happened to be there and to those guys, we looked like easy targets. I felt like even more of a punk because we'd left the girls there. Maybe the guys in rubber masks were just trying to embarrass us in front of the girls or, even worse, bother us for sport.

Technically we were safe, but safety was a relative description as there was no telling how long it would last or what it really meant. Did safety mean that we were free from verbal or physical harm? Did it mean feeling secure and protected? Was safety determined by how resilient one could be in the face of ongoing trauma and violence? Was it all based on perception and expectation?

I wanted to be able to walk around the neighborhood and to the bus stop without feeling like I was a target. I wanted to be able to go to law enforcement because I was being threatened, confident that at least there would be some sort of assessment, investigation, or protection.

Sadly, I didn't feel safe anywhere except inside school or at home in our apartment. I always wondered if the white kids or Asian kids I saw at the track meets had the same feelings. I didn't want to assume what their lives were like in neighborhoods I knew little about—but I knew they'd get chances that my friends and I were unlikely to get. My foster brother Angel, for example, certainly didn't get those chances. Only Black boys were taught (or learned the hard way) that they had to be cautious around the police, rather than seeing them as a source of help. Only Black boys were taught (or again, learned the hard way) to be cautious of random dudes walking around the corner—often dudes who looked like us. Their parents never had to have conversations with them about being cautious when talking to white people, about changing the intonation of your voice and being perceived as a threat. We all knew as Black boys, and later as Black men, that our likelihood of being arrested for anything was higher than our white peers.

The police force in my community operated to flatten the crime rate—not to heal the community or work hand in hand with others to do so. They were there to keep a kind of rough order—and sometimes, as in the case of the cops who didn't help us, not even to do that.

The numbers back up what I was learning by experience. Thirty percent of American Black males had been arrested at least once by the age eighteen as opposed to 22 percent for American white males of the same age; by the age of twenty-three, about 49 percent of Black men had been arrested as opposed to about 38 percent for white men in the same age group.[3] The Black Youth Project Survey found that Black youth reported the highest rate of harassment by the police at 54.5 percent, nearly twice the rate of other young people.[4] Fewer than half of Black youth trust the police, compared with 71 percent of white youth, 59.6 percent of Latino youth, and 76.1 percent of Asian American youth. Substantially fewer Black young people believe the police in their neighborhood are there to protect them, compared to people from other racial and ethnic groups.

What these hard numbers indicate was what I lived every day. Everything around me—the big stories like Rodney King, the incidents in my life like running from those guys and getting no help from the cops—all combined to make me feel that I was unlikely to survive beyond my twenties—that we were all expendable, no matter how well I did in school or on the track. A lot of the young men I work with today feel the same way and are under the same threat. I got out alive and without having to go to prison—but too many don't. Many years later, this part of my young manhood is what led me on my path of working to decrease violence in my community.

CHAPTER 4

GETTING ON TRACK

FROM MY OWN PERSONAL NEED to stay busy and challenge myself and my parents wanting me to stay out of trouble in a productive way, every summer I was enrolled in some sort of academic camp. The camps ranged from computer science, film, music, sports, whatever kept me learning and busy.

At about the age of eleven or twelve, I became interested in architecture. Pratt University, one of the country's premier art, design, architectural, and engineering schools, was just a few blocks from my home. Pratt had a well-designed pre-college summer camp for elementary and high school students. I would eventually spend four summers at Pratt in the camp and precollege programs. My favorite class in the program was called Project Display, which was an introduction to architecture and design. There I learned how to use some of the different architectural drafting tools, do technical drawings, and build my own models to scale.

In the '80s and '90s, there was a big push for Black kids to explore the fields of science, especially engineering and computer science. If you were Black and had decent grades or showed a special interest in STEM (science, technology, engineering, and math), then you were pushed in that direction. I didn't feel pushed though. When I started, I truly wanted to be an architect.

Honestly, Black and Latino representation were needed in every field, other than going to prison. Diversity initiatives went beyond creating future economic opportunities for kids of color; they were vital to the advancement of respective fields. New perspectives and insights that could have never surfaced without BIPOC people in the room had been lost for time immemorial, and structural racism, creating barriers to the sharing of important and potentially transformative ideas coming from kids of color, really ramped up when people began pushing to get us in these doors. For me, it was less about feeling the need to integrate than about getting access to a space and platform to develop ideas that I could bring back home. Frankly, my folks couldn't have cared less about me integrating into an all-white environment, as some sort of poster child, but commonly asked at one of our regular conversations, "What are you going to do when you get into the spaces? How are you going to bring these ideas back home? A lot of kids you know in Brooklyn and in Harlem never get these chances, so how is this going to be different for you? What will you bring back?" They felt strongly that I needed to keep exploring and learning as widely as possible. We were able to manage the summer programs because they were kept affordable.

After a few summers though, I got restless at Pratt. I no longer wanted to go to a program down the street from my high school. Through a friend of my father, I found out about a STEM program, with a focus on engineering at Prairie View A&M University, an HBCU (historically Black college or university) in Prairie View, Texas. I applied and was accepted with full room and board covered. All I needed was to pay for a plane ticket down there.

I'd never been to Texas and had preconceived notions about what to expect. It was the longest plane ride I'd been on by myself and it was thrilling! When I got there, I was a little disappointed that I didn't see anyone walking around in cowboy boots or ten-gallon hats en route to rodeos.

Prairie View was just about an hour outside of Houston and a lot less urban than I'd expected. I'd been in rural places before, but rural upstate New York and rural Texas were very different. I saw fewer mountains and dense tree foliage and canopies, and more open spaces and real prairies with a mixture of dried tall grasses and shrubs with a few scattered trees.

I met Black kids from all over the US but mostly from Texas. Our counselors were college students enrolled at Prairie View, mostly hailing from Texas, but a few were from other states. We studied together and, in our downtime, shared the universal language of hip-hop. We all listened to the Houston-based rap group the Geto Boys, whose single "Mind Playing Tricks on Me" populated radios in both New York City and Texas, and I filled them in on some East Coast artists like Das EFX, Gang Starr, and underground hip-hop mixes from the Awesome Two, which I dubbed from the radio. They introduced me to more Texas rap groups like UGK and Ganksta NIP.

That was the fun part. What was less fun, I realized, was work in engineering. I liked the engineering and design courses, but I wasn't a fan of the required physics classes, or at least how they were taught. Rather quickly, I was beginning to shift away from my earlier ambitions.

I went to Bishop Loughlin Memorial High School (Loughlin for short), a Catholic school in Clinton Hill, after a bumpy middle school period. Prior to Loughlin, my grades had gotten so low that my parents were threatening to send me to military school. I liked wearing army fatigues as part of my aesthetic, but being forced to wear them wasn't so appealing. In an attempt to turn the ship around, I took the test for New York City's specialized science high schools. Here in New York, there are several schools that are incredibly demanding and prestigious, where admittance is determined through one standardized test. I came close enough for one of the science schools, Brooklyn Tech, and was admitted to the school's conditional program. If I performed well there, I'd have gone on to that school. But my head wasn't in school, and I failed the math course and screwed up that opportunity to attend Brooklyn Tech.

That left me out in the cold. I was zoned for Erasmus Hall, an enormous high school that once had a stellar reputation but that was now riddled with gang violence. I did *not* want to go there. The neighborhood kids who went there didn't want to go there either— no one should have to be afraid at school. Erasmus had a reputation for a lot of fights, both in school and out of school, much like many underfunded and overcrowded schools around the US. Intentional violence for any person could cause both emotional and physical pain, but violence experienced as a child, in a person whose brain is still rapidly developing, can have long-term and seriously detrimental consequences. The more ACEs a kid has, the more likely that will impede academic success. These students experienced more problems concentrating in school, had higher school dropout rates, poorer reading skills, and increased aggressive behavior and internalizing of emotions compared to those without ACEs.[1]

Erasmus's graduation level was lower than the US average. Reasons for a student dropping out of any school could include needing to work full time to support their family, lacking social support systems at the school, and being bullied or experiencing some sort of violence at school. According to the National Survey of Children's Exposure to Violence, 37.3 percent of American youth experienced a physical assault from one of their peers or siblings; 67.5 percent of kids surveyed had at least witnessed or had direct experience with some sort of violence, crime, or abuse.[2] Violence experienced as a youth qualifies as an adverse childhood experience. In poor Black and Brown neighborhoods, people usually have more than one ACE.

I had to think of an alternative to Erasmus or military school, a privilege I knew I had and couldn't afford to blow again. Redemption came in the form of Loughlin. After learning about the high school from friends, I applied and they decided to take a chance on me. I'm grateful they did because that's where I really did begin to work harder and more effectively. Before I got to Loughlin, I wasn't headed for the streets exactly—but neither was I headed for my fullest potential. My time at Loughlin and the mindset I developed there helped me reach that potential. I appreciate it to this day.

My parents had to scramble for the tuition money. Catholic schools are not as pricey as elite nondenominational or independent prep schools, but they are a few thousand dollars a year. Knowing that they were trusting me, I thought, *I can't screw this up*. I wanted to reward their sacrifice.

Loughlin's smaller classes helped me to focus and get help when I needed it. But the other thing that helped as much, if not more, was getting onto the track team with my buddies Nigel and Ant. Running served as an outlet for the boundless energy that had made it hard for me to sit still in school. Track burned it off and helped me to focus for long periods of time without struggling. I didn't want to disappoint myself, my coach, or my teammates. And my competitive spirit started to come out, not only in running but in class. I wanted to get better at what I was presented with, whatever it was. I wanted to excel. I started getting up early to study before school and my grades started to inch up. I stayed up late after practice studying. I went to the library on weekends when I wasn't competing in a race. I even made my way into the honors program in a short period of time and remained there until I graduated.

Sure, running hurt—on that first day of working out in Fort Greene Park, I threw up my lunch during the workout and had dry heaves running up and down the steep hills there. I thought to myself, "This shit sucks and I'm not good at this," but in a funny way, that's what kept me going. I don't like being bad at stuff; I wanted to keep doing it so I could improve.

Loving what running was doing for me, I did it more and more and was eager to train all year. So when I learned about the Running School, a cross-country camp in the Catskills, I was game, even though old ankle injuries and sprains left me in pain after running. I was determined to go no matter what—I'd already paid my deposit and had no desire to spend the summer in Brooklyn, sweating and worrying about being jumped.

The Catskill Mountains of New York are beautiful, wooded, and hilly, just a few hours from Brooklyn but, in terms of the atmosphere, a million miles away. It was serene, rural, focused. There were kids at the Running School—maybe two hundred or more—from all over the country, and we were there with one goal, to get stronger as cross-country runners. I liked cross-country and wanted to get better at it, but I wasn't good at it and it really wasn't my field. I just hoped the training would make me a better middle-distance runner during the indoor and outdoor track-and-field season. The Running School was tough whether you liked cross-country or used it for track-and-field conditioning. The coaches expected the best of us and truly ran us ragged. But being out in the fresh air, not having to stop at stoplights, meeting kids with the same goals as me—it was all that I'd hoped for and more. I loved the camaraderie, being with a bunch of kids my age, most of whom I didn't already know, and who didn't have some idea of me from school.

I learned to run in pain but because of the increased mileage at camp, I had to get my ankles taped up before every morning and afternoon run by the sports medicine doctors and athletic trainers, who were very cool. They asked me a lot of questions about my training and injuries and just regular small talk. It didn't take much time for me to feel comfortable asking them questions—partly because I wanted to learn what I might be able to do to expedite my healing but also because what they were doing was interesting to me. They seemed happy in their jobs. How often do you see that? After a while, I got up the nerve to ask if I could see patients with them in my off times and they said I could. Not only did they let me shadow them and observe more closely what they were doing but they taught me about the different types of injuries that runners and athletes experienced and how it impacted their abilities to train and compete. I would be in the clinic for one to two hours a day and toward the end of the week they let me tape up the runners and apply ace bandages around the other injured runners. I began to learn some basic anatomy and, to some extent, how to relate to patients.

With all the different camps and programs I'd been to, I'd spent a number of summers looking at different career possibilities, but that was the first time I'd spent observing someone working, where the people seemed to deeply enjoy what they were doing. The doctors and the trainers were all runners who loved working with runners. They were completely dedicated to helping people heal up so that the patients could get back to the sport that they were so passionate about. I wanted to have that same feeling when I had a job in the future.

When I was a kid and went to the pediatrician, it was just something I had to do to stay healthy. I never thought about the work involved or what it might be like on the other side of the exam table, helping people be healthier. Now I wanted to recreate the feeling I had when I was shadowing the doctors at the Running School, that feeling of being happy at work and helping people in the process. I'll add that none of the docs or trainers were Black. That wasn't a deterrent though—I just liked the work and felt more than capable of learning it.

In 1993, though, that next summer, something else happened that influenced me greatly. I had to see an orthopedic surgeon for my ankle problems and newer knee pain, and he turned out to be a Black man, Dr. Answorth Allen. This jolted me into realizing—and really considering—that most medical professionals were white. At some level, that spurred my desire as well. I had already decided I wanted to become a doctor. Who I was going to become as a doctor was beginning to take shape.

CHAPTER 5

THE SWATS, RED DOGS, AND THE REALITY OUTSIDE THE MOREHOUSE GATES

I HAD AN EARLY ACCEPTANCE LETTER, and I was ready to go. I was moving to Atlanta, Georgia, as an incoming freshman at my dream school, Morehouse College. My trunk had been packed since Thanksgiving, which was also the time I stopped telling people that I was in high school. In my mind, I was already a college student in Atlanta.

When moving day came, I was up early, excited about leaving home and excited about new beginnings. I was being a little obsessive, repeatedly going through my suitcases with my clothes and the rusted trunk Pop bought from one of our regularly frequented second-hand stores downtown Brooklyn to make sure I wasn't leaving behind anything I could potentially need over the next few months. I was staring at my luggage and going through it almost as a meditation. I used it to get into a zone and started focusing on what I was going to be at Morehouse. I knew I wanted to be a leader and change things and was going to somehow do it as a doctor.

I was inspired to apply to and attend Morehouse by my older cousin Jason, who I was partly raised with. He was one of my biggest influences. He ran track, so I ran track. He always seemed to be focused and disciplined about athletics and academics, so I did the same, except for a two-year hiccup during middle school. He went to Morehouse, so I got Morehouse fever. "You can learn at any school," Jason said, "but it's expected that you become a leader if you go to Morehouse." That got to me. The last line of the personal statement of my application to Morehouse read: "When my name is mentioned, would people hold their heads up high or bow their heads in shame?" I wanted to create my own legacy as a leader.

On my first night in Atlanta, I was in my dorm room, flopped on the bed, thinking about upcoming track practice, classes, and life at Morehouse. What was it going to be like? Suddenly, there was a knock at the door. I jumped up, surprised. I didn't think I was going to have a roommate and I didn't know anyone there yet. I opened the door.

"You the cat from New York?" came a loud, fast Southern accent.

"Yeah?" I responded a bit warily.

"I'm Tracy Knox. Coach Hill told me to come get you and show you around. You hungry?" He asked all in one breath. The Atlanta accent was characteristically Southern but spoken extra fast.

"Peace, I'm Rob Gore. Yeah, I'm hungry."

He told me that everybody called him "T Knox." We gave each other a pound and snapped fingers at the end (Southern style) like my friends from Texas had shown me a few years prior.

I was glad T Knox stopped by because I was starving. I was eighteen years old and had a high metabolism and didn't hesitate to grab any opportunity to eat. All I knew about food in Atlanta from a previous visit and the twelve hours I'd been there that day was that I didn't have to ask for sugar in iced tea, grits were a school (and citywide) breakfast staple, and collard greens were available as a side at every restaurant and in the cafeteria.

We headed out of the dorm and got in his Jeep. I was glad to meet somebody who had a car—it was far from standard in New

York City for people my age. OutKast played from the tape deck while I got a tour of the Atlanta University Center (AUC), the largest consortium of Black colleges and universities in the US. It is composed of Morehouse's campus along with other HBCU's nearby, including Morris Brown College, Clark-Atlanta University, Morehouse School of Medicine, Spelman College, and the Interdenominational Theological Center, and was one of the few havens, outside of Africa and the Caribbean, that dedicated itself to the education of Black people. I just stared out the window hypnotized by both the melody and the rolling streets with no traffic but a few old Cutlass Supremes playing a mixture of "booty-shake" music and Southern hip-hop, which was almost nonexistent back home. We drove down Fair Street and James P. Bradley Drive and past "Club Woody," or Woodruff Library, the communal AUC library that was near Clark-Atlanta's campus.

Morehouse was extra special to me because it was the only college in the US that was dedicated to educating solely Black men. And beyond the campus, there was the sense of expanding my world, of not being up north anymore. It manifested in profound ways like realizing that Dr. Martin Luther King had walked the same halls and lived in the same dorms that me and my classmates did, or in seeing the civil rights movement sites that I'd only seen on TV. And then in minor cultural things. I arrived on a broiling hot day in my jeans and long-sleeved shirt, the height of Brooklyn fashion. But I quickly realized I was going to have to stop with my New York antics—this outfit wasn't going to work in the deep Georgia heat.

"If you want to get work done, go to Douglass Hall at Morehouse. Too many women at Club Woody, but there ain't gonna be no distractions at Morehouse," Tracy advised. I just nodded my head politely, though I completely got where he was coming from.

A little way further from the AUC, we pulled up at a Wendy's. At last! I was beyond hungry. We ordered the food, ate immediately, while talking about music, classes we planned to take, running track, and what was to come this year. We were finishing our food when a platoon of soldiers, all Black dudes, wearing all-black fatigues with assault rifles strapped to their sides and guns in holsters, walked in. I was hoping it was just to order food—I was shook. I'd never felt comfortable being in the presence of police, and ones walking around with weapons I'd seen in war movies only accentuated that feeling. "You know who that is?" T Knox whispered. "Those are RED DOGs," he said quietly, trying not to alert the famished death squad. The RED DOGs were a special narcotics police unit in Atlanta whose name stood for "Run Every Drug Dealer Out of Georgia."

The RED DOG Unit was formed in 1989 during the time of the crack epidemic as a way to provide "proactive police presence in areas that have a high incidence of street drug sales, use, and drug-related crimes."[1] They were a paramilitary police unit with special training and had a reputation for being excessively aggressive with the sole purpose of striking fear into drug dealers as well as the general public.

There was no question that areas with high numbers of both drug sales and street drug use had high levels of violence. I understood then the need for people to feel safe in their neighborhood, but people weren't any safer. During the 1980s and 1990s, the war on drugs resulted in massive numbers of incarcerated Black and Brown bodies every year, most often they were the same age as me, the same build as me, faces just like mine being called "public enemy number one."

The paramilitary police were part of an age-old tactic of force and fear that doesn't work. Since 1971, when Richard Nixon declared a "war on drugs," there has been a steady and multipronged escalation in largely ineffective efforts to control the drug trade. The mission of the RED DOGS was to have drug dealers leave the streets of certain parts of Atlanta and its suburbs by whatever means necessary. It made me think that the people in power were OK with crack being used and sold, and even OK with the violence that accompanied the sale, production, and use of drugs—just as long as it didn't happen where they lived. Shifting it out of sight and out of mind allowed the good citizens and authorities in Atlanta not to even try to understand the multidimensional causes of drug abuse or to take any significant steps to address those causes.

All the bullets, Kevlar, and big trucks in the world didn't make Atlanta safer; it just pushed the problem away from one area and deeper into others. Seeing how Atlanta was stricken by crack in the poorest neighborhoods helped me realize that neighborhood problems wouldn't be solved by more cops and more guns. What happened in Atlanta is what so often happens—the cops started to abuse their power. In 2011, a few years after I first saw them in that Wendy's, the RED DOGS were disbanded after a series of out-of-court settlements, including one for reckless abuse of a motorist due to a public strip and search and another for a raid at the Atlanta Eagle, a gay bar where the RED DOGs were said to have hurled homophobic slurs and otherwise abused the patrons.

Seeing the RED DOGs on that first night out in Atlanta was a strong warning that—although I had left New York thinking I was headed some place safer and maybe even a bit of a utopia in Morehouse College—I had landed in the middle of a war zone complete with paramilitary ready to intimidate, in military fashion, a neighborhood of poor people. Even though I was just passing through as a student, most of these people looked like me. The message was clear. Be afraid. Be very afraid.

Still, nothing could take away my joy at being at Morehouse and my happiness at being in Atlanta—or my determination to do well. At Morehouse I continued running cross-country and track and was a biology major. I was intent on becoming a doctor and I didn't want to let my family or myself down by flunking out and having to return home. I wasn't on scholarship—the money came from my folks, some of my relatives, a scholarship from my church, birthday and holiday gifts, and my own summer job savings. I didn't want to waste their money or my own.

And I had one other thing driving me. I started locking my hair at Morehouse but before I got there and made that decision, I had one last haircut from my regular barber. I was so excited to tell him that I was leaving for Morehouse. But instead of congratulating me, he chuckled and said, "Have fun! You'll be back here for good after Christmas." He went on to tell me of some friends who had gone away to college but always ended up flunking out and coming back to Brooklyn without a degree. I'll never understand why he reacted that way. Was he just being a dick? Did he have dreams he'd given up on? Did he feel I was stepping out of place, that I should stay where I had been born and raised? I'll never know. But I damn sure wasn't going to prove him right.

When I wasn't studying or at practice, I thoroughly enjoyed the debates with my classmates about subjects high and low: whose city had the best-looking women, the state of the Black family, theology, hip-hop, and a million other things. It was thrilling to be in the midst of so many remarkable young Black men. It was thrilling to consider I was one of them.

Not all my learning was in the classroom either. As a Brooklynite, I had some preconceived notions about people who spoke with a Southern drawl—I had bought into the stereotype that this person might not be as intelligent as people who come from other places. But in Atlanta I met guys who came from Mississippi and rural Alabama and who had these Southern drawls—and were absolutely brilliant. It was like, wow, I need to open my mind here. My perception of what smart kids sounded like was completely shifted.

I was in honors classes all through middle and high school but in inner-city Brooklyn, there were only a handful of other Black guys in those classes, the majority of the honors students were girls. So to enter an environment of academic excellence where everybody looked like me was different. To see other people the same gender as me, who came from similar communities and who were doing the work became my standard. I realized this utopia of Black excellence could really exist. It became my mission, over time, to spread that vision as far as I can. To this day, more than thirty years later, I wear my Kings County Hospital badge on a Morehouse College lanyard so my patients can see it and so I never forget that pledge and that place.

Premed studies at Morehouse were tough, but I was finding myself increasingly committed to becoming a doctor and I knew I wanted to serve the Black community, both as a role model and as a physician within those communities. I spent most of my time learning and studying inside a building called Nabrit Mapp McBay, named after Drs. Samuel M. Nabrit, Frederick Mapp, and Henry McBay, all of whom had taught science at Morehouse.

I came to know the building well because I was there at least four or five days a week and sometimes more in the G Bio lab. G Bio was short for General Biology, a course required for all science majors. As often happens, many of the guys who started out in the major were planning to be premed, but as time went on, some faded away as they realized health care wasn't for them. My love for the field remained, nurtured by the Health Careers Society, an organization that all the pre-health-professional students had to join. The Health Careers Society was run by Dean Thomas Blocker, the premedical dean and head of the G Bio lab. Dean Blocker, or "Block" when he wasn't around, was a giant of a man, who demanded excellence from every student he came across. "What you say you are, you are now becoming" is what he would regularly say to students at the start of a Health Careers meeting, or whenever he felt it warranted. Over the years Dean Blocker and I would have countless talks, but one that stood out the most was when he said, "Your presence is needed in medicine and you cannot afford to be anything but excellent. Peoples' lives will depend on what you have learned Brother Gore." Excellence had to be achieved.

Health Careers meetings guided students through the ins and outs of applying to medical school and how to study for the Medical College Admissions Test and other standardized professional exams. We also had regular visits from health professionals giving advice about their chosen careers and specialties. We met representatives from summer research and enrichment programs from around the US. Most of the speakers were Black and were often graduates of HBCUs, and they were all excited to come speak with us, on their own time, about their experiences in navigating medicine and health care. It was amazing to hear the stories of incredibly accomplished role models like Dr. Barbara Ross-Lee, the first Black woman dean of a US medical school (at the College of Osteopathic Medicine of Ohio University), and Dr. David Satcher, the first Black US surgeon general, among other distinctions. To have Black women and Black men, many of whom had sat in the same classes, in some of the same buildings, even in some of the same seats that we were currently occupying, was especially inspiring. Health Careers was a gold standard for the type of mentorship and guidance that an organization could offer. I carried those standards with me later when I helped form Minority Medical Student Emergency Medicine (MMSEM), a program that worked to bring more students of color into emergency medicine.

Life on campus was good. But when I left campus, I was transported into a different world, raw and unprotected. Folks in Atlanta called that area the SWATS—short for Southwest Atlanta. It was a mixture of historic buildings and streets named after civil rights heroes, housing tenements, run-down houses, and fast-food spots. Morehouse, as intellectually stimulating as it was, was still in the 'hood. There were two different worlds separated by less than fifty feet of concrete and street. Outside of the hallway window of my dorm I could easily see police car chases, people smoking crack, and transgender sex workers who strolled up and down Ashby Street, which ran parallel to the campus. The wrought-iron gates and brick walls that separated the campus from the community did little to deafen the sounds of police sirens and regular nighttime gunfire that sounded off like crickets in the country. Morehouse's metal gates created a theoretical protection from the outside world but still allowed the smell of burning grease to waft through from Mrs. Winner's Chicken, one of the local fast-food spots across the street from the school—because you could only stay on campus for so long.

I had never seen shacks before. This was in 1994, but just like in old documentaries, movies, and even cartoons about the South, there were still people living in shacks just down the street from the school. Often the people on the porches, Black like me, looked at us like they couldn't relate to us, or maybe they hated us because we were in this ivory tower across the way from them.

It made me uncomfortable to feel separated in the neighborhood I was living in, disconnected from the people who lived there, especially since my main reason for going to Morehouse was to be able to work in and serve neglected and disregarded communities. But fear is powerful, and to be told to stay away from the world beyond the gates of Morehouse or the entire Atlanta University Center, was certainly compelling, but it seemed more like cowering in comfort than building community relationships. It didn't take too long but I began to venture outside of the gates and to work in this close but unfamiliar part of the neighborhood.

I first volunteered with a program called Inner Strength, founded by a friend, fellow Morehouse student, and native New Yorker named Val Joseph whose nickname was "Flow." Inner Strength worked with young Black men in the community just outside Morehouse to provide mentorship and support and to offer alternatives to street life.

I later volunteered with another program called the Children's Breakfast Table (CBT) founded by a Spelman student named Tiffany Hunter, then known as "Uhuru." CBT was patterned after the Black Panther Party's Free Breakfast for Children program, and we cooked and fed breakfast to kids in public housing around Atlanta, many of whom didn't eat regularly. At CBT, I learned the importance of going to where the need was. The weekly breakfasts and kids activities were set up in a community center near the public housing. But just because you have a good idea doesn't mean people will naturally gravitate toward it. In order to build community trust, we walked around the different housing units, knocking on doors to meet the people living there, informing them what we were doing, and inviting them and their children to participate (this was pre–cell phone and very few people had in-house internet). The goal wasn't just to invite kids to breakfast but to build relationships with the people there. If there was a positive relationship built and trust was established, kids came and their caretakers felt supported, which was the goal.

During my spring break, I wasn't able to go back to Brooklyn, but a new volunteer opportunity called the Spring Break Challenge placed Morehouse students at nearby Booker T. Washington High School. Washington High was Atlanta's first Black high school and just a few blocks from campus, up Ashby Street. Interested students at Morehouse who stayed at school during the holiday volunteered to work as tutors and mentors during their week of vacation. Since I couldn't be at home with family because of track practice and limited money, I leapt at the chance to volunteer. I came to feel connected to the work and the students who I met, and I became committed to service at the school, continuing to work at Washington High weekly until I graduated three years later.

There was a kid I worked with, I think his name was Melvin; after all this time, I'm not sure of his name but I still remember his face. He was in the general chemistry class, in his senior year. His teacher asked me to help him with his work because he was having some challenges. Before I started talking to Melvin about neutrons and electrons, which is what the class was learning at the time, I needed to understand who he was and determine what his motivation was for being in school. I needed to establish a quick rapport and build some trust. I asked him, "What do you wanna do when you grow up," and he said, "I wanna be a truck driver." Melvin had this hardcore Atlanta accent, similar to T Knox, and two gold teeth on his bottom canines. He was heavyset, had a slight odor to him, and seemed like he hadn't had a chance to shower for some time. The shirt he wore also looked like it hadn't been washed for a while given the dirt streaks on the arms, front of the shirt and his collar. I didn't know his home life situation and wasn't in a position to ask about it. What I did know was that Washington High was in the SWATs. The SWAT's had large pockets of poverty and 100 percent of the student body were economically disadvantaged. Who could know what other kinds of privations he'd been suffering. After we exchanged pleasantries and chatted for a while, I said, "Let's go over this stuff," and I asked him to read out loud to me. One thing became clear immediately—he couldn't read. He struggled to read basic words that had nothing to do with anything science related. Did he have a learning challenge or had he just never been taught? Obviously, he had just been pushed along and pushed along and pushed along. He was a really pleasant guy and that was probably part of how it happened. One year after another, one bad class after another, and here he was—nearly an adult and illiterate. Unfortunately, Melvin's story wasn't uncommon, but as a college kid it made a huge impression on me. Ever since then, when I'm teaching, I try not to make people feel bad about what they don't know. And I'm always looking for opportunities to teach. But then I was just a college volunteer—I couldn't see him through to literacy, but Melvin's image stayed with me. He wasn't necessarily a victim of violence per se, but clearly a victim of another kind of neglect. I couldn't be sure about his situation, but it was obvious that while he was being shuffled along, the services he needed weren't being provided. Childhood adversity like poverty and limitations to formal education impacted how long people stayed alive. People with bachelor's and master's degrees had a higher life expectancy than those with only a high school diploma. Compared to people living above the poverty level, poor people had a lower life expectancy.[2] How would Melvin be able to do anything beyond survive?

There were always students getting robbed walking from the MARTA (Atlanta's train system) late at night. They carried shopping bags from department stores in the Lennox and Phipps Malls, while exposing their one or two skinny gold chains around their necks for people to see and admire. I didn't really feel bad for them because I thought they should know better walking past the projects before getting to campus with an almost neon sign inviting someone to rob them. I did recognize that not all the students thought about safety or had a sense of impending doom since some of them grew up in gated and affluent urban and suburban cities where watching your back was something done only by characters on TV. Death, however, was different. It was permanent. Clothes, sneakers, and jackets could be repurchased. Even the anxiety that occurred initially or after being robbed could possibly get better with time and with the resources for good counseling, but there was no return from death. And death came calling.

A few months into my first year, three Morehouse students were killed in random acts of violence: George Moore, a freshman like me, from Wilmington, Delaware, was shot and killed while he was driving by one of the projects in the city. A few weeks later, Oronde Bell, a student from Roxbury, Massachusetts, was shot dead by a carjacker not far from the campus. The very same week, yet another Morehouse man, Michael Singleton, was shot and killed in an off-campus housing robbery. I didn't know the exact circumstances around their murders but that didn't make me feel any better. I didn't want to call home and talk to my folks about it out of fear that they might make me move back to Brooklyn.

Atlanta was a city of civil rights heroes, affluence, poverty, and an increasing number of homicides, a reminder that the work of the civil rights movement was far from done. A reminder that trying to unsee or escape a community under siege—rather than developing an understanding of it—would be part of the travesty and the sin of "low aim" that Dr. Benjamin Elijah Mays, Morehouse president emeritus and mentor to Dr. King, had spoken of.

There was an expectation that students made mistakes, partied, flunked classes, got better, got serious, and eventually graduated, but college students weren't expected to be killed at the hands of another person. That was something we students perceived that happened to the locals, the same people we looked at through the openings in the campus gates, the ones we passed by on our way to the MARTA station or who worked behind the counters of the fast-food places we frequented. But the travesty of it was our disillusion. We were all Black and the same crimes that claimed them claimed us; the only difference was that our elite position provided a fictitious sense of protection. The SWATS were Black neighborhoods and had pockets of both wealth and poverty, the perfect set up for any sort of heinous crime, resulting in the loss of life. The three murdered students—Oronde, George, and Michael—all came from predominantly Black cities, where the majority of those caught in violence looked like them. The SWATS were no different, despite our expectation of protection solely because we were college students now. And then there were efforts, such as the one I took part in, to reach across that divide, but it never was wholly crossed. More would need to be done.

Every year, every month, and often every day at Morehouse, I was learning, both in and outside of classrooms and labs. I saw the racial, ethnic, and class divides that pervaded Atlanta, and reflected divides all over our country and—as I would come to learn—all over the globe. I lived among young Black men and worked with even younger Black kids and other people of color, many living at, or below, federal poverty lines. I was experiencing the realities of adversity—all the scars of actual violence and the fear of violence, always, but also everyday lack of opportunity, the tyranny of low expectations, the ache of simply having less. And high among those deprivations was quality, compassionate health care. That part, at least, I was more determined than ever to address head-on.

CHAPTER 6

RUFF BUFF AND THE PRICE OF DISINVESTMENT

MOREHOUSE HELPED MAKE the me the man I am today. The wisdom of all the men before me and the men I met while there, and of the women of the AUC, stays with me still and will for the rest of my days. But when it came time for medical school, I made the big decision to step out of the world I'd known, into one that was both familiar and not. After a lifetime of majority Black and Latino schools, I decided to attend what I call a "majority" school—one with predominantly white students. I wanted to jar myself out of my comfort zone (receiving instate tuition didn't hurt). And by choosing medical school at the State University of New York (SUNY) Buffalo, I was both stepping out and returning to the place I was born.

Though my parents moved to Brooklyn when I was four, I was born on the East Side of Buffalo; my mother's family had been there for roughly six generations, and we visited often as I grew up. My parents met there after my mother returned to Buffalo for graduate school and when my father left Chicago to do community work as a conscientious objector to the Vietnam War. My great-great-great-grandfather Benjamin Taylor was an abolitionist and the city's first Black physician, a tradition I was proud to continue.

In its heyday, Buffalo's economy was driven by its proximity to a booming steel industry. One of Buffalo's suburbs was Lackawanna, home of Lackawanna Steel, once a major steel producer for the country. People from all over the area made a decent living working there. But like most heavy industry in the US, production began to decline after the 1950s. In 1982, the factory closed, laying off thousands and gutting the local economy.

In med school I lived on the East Side of the city, upstairs from my mother's sister, my aunt Vonnie. In the 1950s and '60s, and even up through visits during my early childhood in the '80s, the East Side was a bustling all-Black neighborhood, a mix of academics, industrial workers and white-collar workers. I thought it was an affluent suburb, but it was just a well-tended part of the city. But by the time I returned for medical school, the thriving neighborhood I knew as a kid was long gone. Still, my grandparents left their Jackson Heights, Queens, apartment and moved back to Buffalo right before I started med school, and still lived there, just a few minutes from my apartment. On my drives to visit them, I saw street after street riddled with dilapidated, boarded-up houses interspersed with homes where people still lived. It was a neighborhood-sized checkerboard of buildings in the stages of life, decay, and desolation.

First in my borough of Brooklyn, then in the SWATS neighborhood in Atlanta around Morehouse and now in Buffalo, I saw the costs of disinvestment, poor education, and untreated trauma every day.

The med school grind was very real and even more intense. I studied a lot at Morehouse, but med school forced me to take it to another level. The amount of material covered in a semester in college was a week's worth of work in medical school. There was very little time to socialize except between classes, during a quick dinner or lunch break, or a special occasion. Every minute of the day had to be accounted for. And the stress of studying was matched only by the stress of feeling lonely and isolated. I liked and got along with the majority of my classmates. They were friendly, but I felt out of place. I'd left Atlanta, a mecca for Black students, as many have called it, and come to a place that was void of them, at least at the school. There were three Black guys in my class, six Black women, three Latino guys, and one Native American out of about 140 students. For some of the other folks of color, who had always gone to majority white institutions, that was the norm. Was this supposed to be accepted because it was the norm? As much as I wanted to dedicate more time to thinking about creating a more diverse med school, I knew that if I flunked out there would be even fewer Black folks in the class, and it might diminish the chances of the school taking another student who looked like me. So I put pressure on myself, but the culture piled it on as well.

The first two years of medical school, the preclinical years, were spent in lecture halls and classrooms, understanding the fundamentals of how the body worked in its normal state and in an unhealthy state. I saw patients every other week in my Clinical Practice of Medicine (CPM) course and spent time in both the outpatient clinics and hospitals. CPM was a nice break from sitting in a classroom and helped to ensure students could make connections with people in the community, effectively communicate with them, and correlate what was being studied and how it related to them and their patients. However, the bulk of time was spent studying, reading, and more reading. I learned intricate details of cell biology, physiology, biochemistry, gross anatomy, neurology, pathology, microbiology, pharmacology, and more for exams, always hoping I would use the material someday to help patients. There was never enough time in the day to study, so after class was over I typically stayed around campus studying, working out, and eating dinner there. I saved time by not driving back and forth from school to home, but I also stayed on campus because it was quiet—and because I didn't have to worry as much about my safety. The hypervigilance I had learned in childhood was still much needed.

I liked my apartment, even though I spent very little time there, beyond eating and sleeping. When I was there, the dysfunction just outside my walls was ever present. I didn't like to be in my neighborhood because it looked abandoned. It was a place that was forgotten about, and the sounds of gunshots at night were kind of distracting while reading. I frequently heard sirens as well, which could have been cops or ambulances. Either way it was a clear indication that someone was having a bad night.

As the years of medical school progressed, I spent more time with patients in the different hospitals and clinics around Buffalo. I was now a third-year medical student wearing scrubs on call days, or shirt and tie on clinic and regular days with my short white coat and feeling like I was really becoming a doctor. It was challenging and different, talking with patients in greater depth, learning more about taking personal and medical histories, studying them, comforting them, and learning from them about their diseases, illnesses, injuries, and the worlds they lived and worked in, hoping the information I was gathering and documenting might eventually save their lives. The classroom learning of the first two years was no longer theoretical. These were real people who happened to be patients, with real problems that were in front of me. Crohn's disease, lupus, HIV and AIDS, asthma, COPD, depression, schizophrenia, tuberculosis, all types of cancer, the list went on and on. Some patients looked pretty good and felt pretty good and came in to the clinics more for the maintenance of their health conditions, kind of like a car tune-up and oil change. Others were rushed to the hospital by car or ambulance to be cared for emergently, ultimately being admitted. The sirens of the night now had a different meaning to me, not just noise, but people in distress, hoping to feel better or live a little longer.

One night, as I ate a late dinner, emergency lights reflecting off the white snow outside brightened up my living room and there was a lot of yelling. I looked out my window to see the commotion; the cops were raiding the dilapidated crack house next door and my neighbor was being escorted out with his hands cuffed and officers pointing guns at his back. It was effed up either way. I don't know what was worse—somebody selling crack next door or a Black man going to prison. I just went back to eating my dinner and continued to study before going to bed. I couldn't even dwell on it because I had more studying to do and needed to be up at 4:30 a.m. to head to the hospital. My white and Asian classmates never saw or spoke about shit like this on their streets, but they didn't live in my neighborhood either. Unfortunately, this was normal for the East Side of Buffalo and its people, many of whom—including my aunt and other family members who stayed because it was the home they knew and loved—couldn't escape the harsh realities around their homes.

A few days after that, while on call, I saw a gunshot wound up close for the first time. I was seven months into my third year and on my general surgery rotation at the Erie County Medical Center (ECMC), Buffalo's public hospital, when the sounds of the multiple trauma pagers in our tiny call room roused our trauma team from a semi-deep sleep in the middle of the night. The general surgery team at the ECMC was also the trauma team, composed of an attending physician, a senior resident, two interns, and me, the medical student, at the bottom of the totem pole. Any patient who had experienced a major injury, whether intentional or accidental, and who risked serious complications from their injuries or immediate death, warranted a trauma evaluation. We hustled to the resuscitation room of the emergency department, where I saw the frightened patient. He had been shot somewhere on the East Side, not far from the hospital or from where I lived. He was close to my age, trembling and tearful, and I couldn't tell if his reaction was due to the pain from his injuries, the cold temperature of the resuscitation room, or the fear that he might die. I trembled as well, feeling my privilege by simply not being the man on the stretcher, but I deeply empathized with him, especially since we were the only two Black people in the room. I had been scared when I was younger, getting hassled and jumped in my neighborhood and seeing a lot of racial hatred all around me in the larger world. But I'd also been lucky. I had the support I needed to make my way out and to make my way through med school and beyond. What might he have been capable of if things were different?

There were more than fifteen of us—doctors, nurses, ER techs, and cops—in the large resuscitation room, crowding around the patient, each with a different role. Though frightened and bleeding, he was still able to speak, and he was quizzed about his personal history and the sequence of events that led to the shooting. For the most part, the medical staff asked questions in a compassionate tone, but the cops were harsher and more confrontational.

I stood to the side of the room, attempting to stay clear of the traffic. Then Dr. Dilip Dan, my senior surgery resident, signaled for me to come by his side to examine the patient's abdomen. A gunshot wound to the anterior abdomen was an automatic indication to go to the operating room to do an "ex-lap," or exploratory laparotomy, to inspect the inside of the abdomen, identify any injuries, and repair them.

The holes in the man's abdomen were small, scantily bleeding, and seemed insignificant at first glance. But I had learned that that was deceptive. Even if a bullet makes a small entry wound, it doesn't always travel in a straight line. Depending on the caliber and where the bullet hits, it can wreak havoc far beyond what's apparent. Dr. Dan had me place my hand on the young man's abdomen to palpate it as part of the exam. His abdomen was firm and he flinched with very minimal pressure. Although the location of the man's injuries indicated he was going to need emergent surgery, the bedside ultrasound also showed there was fluid in the abdomen, another sign there was a significant amount of blood in the abdomen.

Within a few minutes, the patient was intubated and taken to the operating room. In the OR Dr. Flynn, the trauma surgery attending, and Dr. Dan quickly opened up the abdomen with a scalpel and bovie, which operates at very high heat, cauterizing and producing the smell of burning flesh. My job was to retract the skin to keep the abdominal cavity more visible while the intestines and other organs were evaluated. After a couple of hours, the surgery was finished. The man on the table survived.

Even after the emergency had been over for a few hours, I wasn't sure what I was supposed to feel. I was still anxious but couldn't pin it to residual adrenaline or some form of fear. On one hand I was happy and excited that the patient was still alive, but on the other hand it felt weird that I was smiling like I won some kind of game. The surgeons and nurses seemed like they were all

OK with what had just happened, like it was just in a day's work. I never asked the other surgeons how they felt or how they coped with seeing trauma beyond the science of caring for the patient. I wanted to ask, Was I supposed to feel like this? Was it OK to be anxious or excited about what happened? If the patient was white would you show different sets of emotions or would you tuck them away and compartmentalize them because it's hard to perform and think straight if you're being emotional? I thought it was exciting to be in a surgery, focusing on every intricate movement being performed. But no one talked about the case after it was over, aside from the details of the surgery. As a med student, you're supposed to be both happy to be in surgery and to learn, but not you're not supposed to draw too much attention to yourself or ask a lot of questions—unless someone asks *you*. Talking about how we felt seemed to break the code and protocol of how doctors dealt with emergencies. I never really questioned whether I was supposed to feel a certain way. I just went along with the program, following the lead of the docs I was working with.

I went home after the morning sign-out rounds around 8 a.m., ate some oatmeal while sitting on the couch, and went to bed to rest for another long day at the hospital. As a physician, you must develop a hard carapace to be able to do what needs to be done—cut into bleeding bodies, cause pain in an effort to cure, tell people terrible news. The best doctors don't develop a hard heart. The compassion needs to remain. But compartmentalizing emotions, at least for a moment, seemed part of the job. That night was my first real lesson in how to do that. But the question that plagued me then—how was I supposed to feel and act seeing someone who could have been me, could easily have been my foster brother, close to death? And what should I have done next? I wasn't going to figure those answers out for a good long time, but from that moment, I could sense that I would need to, sooner rather than later.

Like a lot of med students, I found surgery to be primarily technical—you were the repair person who fixed broken things in the body but not the one who took care of anything beyond the patient's presenting injury. Though I found trauma surgery exciting and interesting, I didn't have a love of being in the OR all the time. Standing in one place for hours while operating lost its appeal as my mind started to drift to other places. I did, however, like spending time in the emergency department and being part of the preliminary resuscitation efforts of patients with different emergencies. By the end of my third year, I decided I was going to into emergency medicine.

The time spent in the emergency department was never dull. It complemented my personality quirk of having trouble sitting still while working. I found it refreshing that the emergency docs I worked with were open about not knowing something and didn't make you feel bad about being ignorant about the patient's problems. They were, however, intent on figuring out what was necessary, whether comfortable or not, to keep their patients alive. It was possible as an emergency physician to develop a mastery of managing and treating emergencies but, because of the plethora of cases seen in the emergency department, it was impossible to develop expertise in every ailment that came through the door. It was common to hear an emergency doc say, "I don't know what this is, but let's look it up and see if we can figure it out together."

When deciding on a specialty to go into, there is an unwritten expectation that you demonstrate your commitment in going into it. That commitment sometimes goes beyond doing a six- to twelve-week rotation in that field. The commitment can often come in the form of working on a project or doing research in that field. After my decision to go in to emergency medicine, one of the people I reached out to was Dr. Ron Moscati. Dr. Moscati was a facilitator in my Scientific Basis of Medicine course, which was our small-group learning course where we explored different medical cases to understand everything about the disease—from the molecular level to physical manifestations, epidemiology, treatment, and prevention. He was excited to hear about my decision to go into emergency medicine and asked if I was interested in doing some research with him and his fellow researcher, Dr. Brooke Lerner. As the head of emergency medicine research for the department, he had a host of projects, but one that stood out was focusing on intimate partner violence, formerly known as domestic violence. He would often say that for every disease or health problem that existed, there was a cause, especially types of violence. But in order to better understand and treat the causes we have to understand who is being impacted, how they are impacted, what is being done and *identify what hasn't been done* as a portal to further fix or eradicate a health issue. I didn't know much about intimate partner violence, but I learned about it over the course of the next year, and it got me thinking more about the patients who came in as victims of intentional violence, like that young man I had seen with gunshot wounds a few months before. Not just treating the problem but developing an understanding of the problem to prevent it, became a personal mantra, even if a lot of what people perceived of emergency medicine involved placing Band-Aids on problems.

I became more and more drawn to emergency medicine, which offered the opportunity to actually save lives and maybe, just maybe, to interrupt cycles of trauma and violence, to actually play a positive role in patients' lives—not just as the one who stitched them back together but as someone who tried to help them go on to stitch the pieces of their own lives back together as well.

There was another reason I felt like I needed to be in the emergency department. One of the main reasons I had for becoming a physician was to practice in Black neighborhoods and other underserved communities. Since most of my rotations in medical school were spent at ECMC, the public hospital, the majority of patients I saw were Black; on the other hand, I hadn't seen any Black emergency medicine docs in Buffalo. I saw a sprinkling of Black docs in the primary care specialties but none in emergency medicine. During my time in the emergency department, or really any place around the hospital, regardless of whether I was taking care of them or not, I was called by many of the Black patients to come to them. Some told me they were in pain and hoped I could help get them medication; some seemed scared and just wanted to talk. I'd hear them talk about their medical problems, including everything from their injuries to abdominal pain to hemorrhoids, but there was a lot of talk of fear and feeling like people didn't understand them or truly heard them. The patients would ask my opinion about getting tests like a CT scan, or whether I thought the medication they were prescribed would really help them or was it some bullshit. I didn't have most of the answers to their questions since I was only a medical student, but their apprehension was a clear indication that they were not comfortable with the care they were receiving. They weren't receiving bad care and I couldn't detect any particular malice, but I could tell there were things that weren't clearly communicated—and better communication might have eased the discomfort they experienced. I know the reason I was pulled aside to talk to them was because I was Black and had a white coat in a place where that was rare. My own family and the friends of my family complained about doctors not paying attention to their needs or feeling like guinea pigs for doctors to try things out on that they would never try on their own family. There's a lot written about the distrust built over the centuries between the medical establishment and Black people—a distrust that was amply justified by the treatment of Black folks not only during the era of slavery but for many decades after. So could it be any wonder that these Black patients, lying vulnerable and afraid for their lives, would want to see a Black medical authority? This issue of experimentation has been well documented in books like *Bad Blood* by James H. Jones about the Tuskegee Syphilis Experiment, Harriet Washington's *Medical Apartheid: The Dark History of Medical Experimentation on Black Americans from Colonial Times to the Present*, and Rebecca Skloot's *The Immortal Life of Henrietta Lacks*.[1]

The Tuskegee Experiment refers to the story of Black men living in Tuskegee, Alabama, who had contracted syphilis and were untreated over decades to see how the disease would manifest over time. The study was conducted by the United States Public Health Service (USPHS) from 1932 to 1972.[2] When the study began, there was no confirmed treatment for syphilis. By the 1940s, though, penicillin had become the gold standard for treatment, and its use reduced rates of syphilis by 75 percent.[3] However, the 399 poor Black men who had contracted the disease and were being studied in Tuskegee were not offered treatment—even though they were led to believe they would be treated for "bad blood," the term for a range of medical problems. The USPHS rationalized there would never be another chance to study the disease in an untreated group like this again. The men of the Tuskegee Experiment wouldn't be offered treatment until the 1970s.

Henrietta Lacks was a Black woman treated for cervical cancer in Baltimore, Maryland, at Johns Hopkins University in the early 1950s. Mrs. Lacks died in 1952, but the tissue biopsy from the tumor on her cervix was found to have properties that allowed the cells to replicate and stay alive a lot longer than other tissue used in science. Her cells were considered "immortal" and were named HeLa cells, the first human cells grown in a culture medium.[4] These cells have been included in over seventy-five thousand scientific studies around the world and have been used to help create the polio vaccine and treatments for the flu, different types of cancer, Parkinson's disease, and HIV, to name a few. However, Mrs. Lacks's cells were taken from her and given to researchers without her or her family's consent and have benefited countless biotech corporations around the world. The case of Mrs. Lacks has led to even greater discussions regarding the ethics of medical consent for treatment and research, specifically among Blacks and other marginalized groups.[5] Stories like these were well known in the Black communities around the country and understandably served to increase suspicion and rejection of medical care by white physicians.

I recalled a conversation I recently had with Dr. Thea James, one of my mentors from undergraduate school. She was the first Black emergency medicine physician I'd worked with and would be the only one I worked with until I would do a rotation at Kings County Hospital in Brooklyn. I'd met Dr. James during an undergraduate premed summer program at the Boston University School of Medicine. She gave me my first exposure to emergency medicine before I started medical school. Dr. James was an attending physician at Boston City Hospital, the public hospital in Boston, similar to ECMC. One afternoon another student named EC Bell and I shadowed her. Like me, EC was a student at an HBCU—Tougaloo College in Jackson, Mississippi. Dr. James was working in a lower acuity section of the emergency department but had me and EC go into the trauma area with another attending physician. While we were there, a Black man in his early twenties, just a few years older than us, came in by ambulance with stab wounds in the left lower quadrant of his abdomen. He was clearly scared and had the same look as the patients I saw at ECMC. Aside from me, EC, and the patient, all of the people who swarmed into the resuscitation room were white. While meeting with Dr. James recently about my decision to go into emergency medicine and inquiring about some guidance in applying to residency, I reflected on that afternoon in Boston with her in the ER several years prior. She told me, "Your presence is needed in the ER! Who else is going to take care of our people?" She was right. Underrepresented docs are more likely to practice in underserved communities than their white peers.[6] I needed to be there not just to diagnose illnesses and give medications but to be an advocate in a way I was now beginning to understand. My presence needed to be even greater.

Some senior physicians from other specialties raised the concern that if I worked in the emergency department, I might miss being able to follow up with patients in the same way they did. They continued to suggest that building lasting doctor-patient relationships came from caring for someone over the course of years. But the fact was that some of the emergency department patients came back so regularly that they felt like family. Unfortunately, the emergency department couldn't resolve their problems. Substance abuse, mental illness, and chronic medical problems required resources beyond the scope of the ED. But what the ED could provide and what was often needed was just a kind word and help alleviating the pain of living, even if it was just a warm bed, a sandwich, some vitamin-infused IV fluids to combat dehydration and intoxication, or maybe a familiar, sympathetic face.

By carefully observing what went on in the emergency department, I began to recognize, on an intuitive level, the various parameters that affect safety and personal and environmental well-being on a societal level. I would later learn that what I was understanding more in depth were social determinants of health— the various conditions that impacted overall health and well-being.

The US Department of Health and Human Services defines "social determinants of health" (SDOH) as "the conditions in the environment where people are born, live, learn, work, play, worship and age that affect a wide range of health, functioning and quality-of-life outcomes and risks."[7] A disease or healthcare issue is seldom the result of one isolated event but rather a series of interconnected events. These conditions and events are influenced by the amount of education a person has, their income, and social support. They are impacted by the physical environment one lives in (which, in turn, is heavily influenced by education and then job access, beginning with safety considerations, as well as exposures to environmental pollutants). SDOH also include the accessibility of healthcare services, as well as the easy access to fresh, unprocessed foods and to sidewalks and parks, which are conducive to exercise and thus help manage and maintain optimal health.

This is a scholarly way of saying that where you live, what biases you face, how much money you have, what life skills you're taught, and how much violence you witness or participate in largely determines how healthy—or unhealthy—you are until the day you die. And for those who don't have enough education or job opportunity, who are forced to accept cheaper housing in unsafe and environmentally unsound neighborhoods, that death is far more likely to be premature.

Specifically, the CDC lists the social determinants of health as the following: healthcare access and quality, education access and quality, social and community context (meaning the strength of community institutions), economic stability, and the neighborhood and built environment (including structural conditions like the availability of sidewalks, grocery stores, and playgrounds). In parts of Brooklyn, in the SWATs (Atlanta), and now in Buffalo, it was painfully obvious to me that without these strong pillars in place, the likelihood of violence escalated enormously. This motif would reoccur as I moved forward in my career, on to Chicago's Cook County Hospital and then back to Kings County Hospital in Brooklyn. I saw it over and over. But I couldn't yet see how I might be a wedge. I was still finding my own way.

My future practice of treating patients in the utmost emergent states had to be balanced with more than a general understanding of how the limits of access to health care, food, education, equitable economic opportunity, and even social support systems within families and the local community impacted all who lived in a community. Buffalo was a petri dish that grew the diseases that happen when you mix limitations in education, poor urban planning, and inadequate economic development in poor communities. My experience was and has been witnessing these substandard conditions only in poor Black communities—but they can occur anywhere there are unmet needs and neglect.

In later years, as I traveled to work in crisis areas in Haiti, Kenya, and other parts of the world, I would see that this formula spelled terrible outcomes for underserved communities of all races, ethnicities, and cultures. For now, it was sinking in as a key lesson for my work as a doctor in the US. And soon enough, I had my long white coat and needed to find a new home to complete my residency.

CHAPTER 7

TO TREAT SUFFERING, KNOW SUFFERING

I DIDN'T SLEEP MUCH at all that first night in the dorms. I tossed and turned in the unfamiliar dark room, occasionally staring up at the ceiling. I was jet lagged, and the hallucinogenic effect of sleep deprivation made me nauseated. The sleep that eventually came was active and intense. Dream-filled sleep that twists sheets off the mattress and tosses a pillow on the floor. I still somehow managed to stay under the mosquito net. Even when I was young, I've found that the battles I fight in my dreams can help me prepare for those I encounter when I wake up. I could have been fighting ninjas or being chased around Brooklyn by goons, which sounds more like practice than a nightmare. The only thing I did remember from that night was weird-looking swirls of color and paisley. It was like a psychedelic trip that I'd seen in movies. I wasn't high, but I did take chloroquine for malaria prophylaxis, which is known to induce vivid and strange dreams.

I was in Nairobi, Kenya, on a two-month elective rotation at the end of medical school to help give me a better understanding of global health and how health care is practiced in resource-limited places around the world. I also wanted to travel and get away before I was to start a grueling residency in July.

I had always wanted to go to Kenya. My mother spent a year studying at the University of Nairobi in the 1960s, shortly after the country had gained independence from Britain. She showed me pictures and souvenirs of her trip and spoke highly and proudly about what it was like being in a place that was mostly Black, not just being in a Black neighborhood. The country was the prototype for an HBCU.

My time in Nairobi was mostly spent at Kenyatta National Hospital (KNH), the biggest hospital in Kenya and one of the largest public hospitals in the world. I spent a significant amount of time doing in-patient practice at KNH's pediatric hospital.

It was a modern-looking building: a grayish block, more functional than aesthetically pleasing, and with windows open for ventilation. Upon entering and walking up the stairs into a long set of dimly lit corridors, I saw a sea of Black and Brown faces expressing a wide range of emotions. Many of the patients were dressed in pale-green hospital pajamas. Some appeared to be fed up with their respective illnesses, waiting impatiently to leave but without any real knowledge of when that day would come. Other patients were outwardly stoic about their condition, no matter how serious it was.

I navigated through groups of mothers wearing brightly colored wraparound dresses and their matching baby carriers with tiny infants strapped to their backs, past countless more Brown and Black faces donning the long and short white coats of the medical staff. Some of the people in white coats were Indian or from the Middle East, but the majority were Black. It was so different from the hospitals in Buffalo, or any other hospital I'd been in, outside of Kings County Hospital in Brooklyn. Aside from the historically Black medical schools that were still open like Howard University in Washington, DC, Meharry Medical College in Nashville, or Charles Drew University in Los Angeles, this was the highest concentration of Black folks I'd ever seen on *either* side of the patient/doctor relationship.

When the Kenyan medical students and I first arrived at Ward 3D, one of the pediatric wards, we all had the same nervous look: a tart mixture of excitement and fear that most medical students have when they first land in clinical rotations. It's a fear of *not* knowing. One of the most unsettling things for medical students who are smart and driven is to remain in a perpetual state of ignorance. Even before medical school, as a premed student, your whole world orbits around your ability and preparation.

Most medical students I've met are driven, focused, and filled with purpose. Make no mistake: being focused on the goal of becoming a competent doctor, to best take care of your future patients, is a powerful tool in medicine, and so is having excellent study habits. But working with patients requires confidence that you will not find in any book. This kind of self-control amid chaos is often lacking in even the best students because of a disconnect between what they spent the last four years reading about and the mantle of responsibility growing on their shoulders. As a physician, you are subject to the fear of not knowing what's going to come through the door. Even with the sum of your practice, your mistakes, and your experiences as a student, the stress you feel each time you walk into a new situation is different. You're not protected by the classroom setting.

There is an ocean of information to master before a physician can provide quality patient care. We all sported the "fake it till you make it" face to keep from crying or buckling under the pressure. Becoming that physician with a fluid way of taking a patient's history, having a calming effect on whatever situation we walked into, *and* a profound level of efficiency was what we all aspired to. I was far from that level in Kenyatta National but was hoping my breakthrough would happen any minute.

Learning, studying, practicing, and continuing to read all the books suggested by more senior doctors seemed the best option. Learning to trust the process was a process in itself. One had only to look into the eager and slightly fearful eyes of medical students to separate us from the more confident residents and attending physicians.

Ward 3D in the hospital had five large rooms, some with multiple beds and cribs on each side, others just beds. Each room was dedicated to housing patients with specific illnesses and ages. There was a room with infants and toddlers who had common colds and respiratory infections, one for patients with hematologic problems like sickle cell anemia or thalassemia, and so on.

Space was a precious commodity at KNH, and sometimes patients were placed wherever there was free occupancy, even if it meant that very sick children had to share beds with children who were less so. It wasn't much different for the mothers and caretakers either. Adjacent to the cribs and beds were multiple long sheets of cardboard on the floor, serving as makeshift beds for the mothers to sleep on. I don't remember seeing any techs or nursing assistants on the ward, so the mothers were the ones cleaning, feeding, and caring for their children during the admission. Some of the mothers were breastfeeding; others fed their children mushy cereal, which oozed from the sides of their mouths and dripped down the front of their gowns. Exhausted mothers slept on the floor motionless. I don't recall ever seeing a father on the pediatric ward, nor did I see any male caretaker sleeping on a piece of cardboard next to their sick child.

When a kid was obviously feeling better, they would jump and move around, smile and coo, but I never saw the mothers smile. It could have been anything: the triple occupancy beds their children had to sleep in, being upset their children were sick, the deep concern of whether their child would get better or not, sleeping on the floor, or the sadness of poverty. The mothers never argued about the deplorable and unfit conditions they and their children were in. It was accepted, but I couldn't help but speculate if the substandard environment was tolerated because there was nothing they had to compare their experiences and current circumstances to. I would have raised hell if this was what I had to endure within my own country, but I had something to compare it to.

Strictly speaking, the hospitals were only there to diagnose, identify, and provide necessary treatments for their patients. All the caregiving was the responsibility of the families, both in the hospital and once they were discharged. In the US, nurses and aides do the majority of the in-hospital caregiving, almost always feeding and bathing their patients.

Some of the kids didn't look too sick based on my limited insight, but there were many kids who were malnourished, which was heartrending to see. There were the kids with swollen legs and distended bellies suffering from kwashiorkor, a type of malnutrition caused by inadequate protein in the diet but adequate calorie intake. This typically occurs when all the child has to eat is rice or corn, nothing else. Others, who were emaciated, with their bones almost completely visible but covered by their skin, had marasmus. Marasmus was similar to kwashiorkor, but these children were in this state because of insufficient calories from any source of food or having nothing to eat at all.

The young children were warriors and fighting to hold onto whatever vitality they had in them. They had shells for bodies with sunken eyes and frail limbs, too weak to feed themselves but taking in nutritional supplements with the aid of a mother, or sister or aunt, helping feed them with a spoon and with the added assistance of intravenous fluids.

I felt sick being there. I felt sick about my privilege. Some of the injuries, diseases, and medical conditions seemed so far removed from any reality I'd previously known. This was something I read in textbooks and saw in commercials with white folks talking about donating money to sponsor a Black or Brown kid somewhere in the developing world, but here it was real. It wasn't a commercial. These kids were dying from not having enough to eat, and back home in the States, food was wasted daily or overly consumed.

Being there went beyond reflecting on grand inequities of race, power, and abundance. Being in the zeitgeist of the problem went further than consuming any amount of the stereotypical imagery of the suffering of people of color—dirty and dying in some distant land. Dr. Frantz Fanon articulated it best when he said, "The poverty of the people, national oppression and the inhibition of culture are one and the same thing."[1] This went well beyond my patients not having enough to eat or even being born poor. Their clinical reality was a reflection of the systemic poverty brought about by another group's pursuit of power and dominance.

These inequities, drawn along the lines of pigment and language, wouldn't have existed had it not been for European colonization of the African continent. Things got precipitously worse after colonial turning points like the 1884 Berlin Conference, which divided the African continent among well-provisioned foreign invaders like the British, the Dutch, and the Portuguese.[2] European powers, by screwing up natural boundaries, pushed natural enemies into the same spaces, bringing about an unnatural competition, and disrupting cohesion among the peoples of Africa. And needless to say, the colonial powers encouraged the enmity among local ethnic groups since it made controlling them much easier. This forced a cycle of trauma to develop on the continent and set the tone for the system of oppression that ultimately made my presence in Kenya so vital. What I was seeing with the patients was only one small part of the result of a much larger problem.

The thoughts in my head swayed back and forth from empathy to frustration, birthed of sheer sensory overload. I was overwhelmed trying to manage and understand the physical ailments the kids experienced, the social system of poverty, the history of colonialism in their lives, while, as a scientist, trying to grasp the best clinical way to treat the conditions I was seeing. The questions of why I was seeing this and the how this continued to happen stood like a heavy shadow behind every patient I cared for. And the answers to those questions couldn't easily be compartmentalized, nor should they.

There was a responsibility to understand the root cause in these cases of their misery. This was the responsibility of any caregiver. If not, then the efforts of caring for patients were doomed, whether intentionally or subconsciously, to keep that person and all their peers suffering in that same space and condition. If I was truly going to contribute to fixing social inequities, whether it be in Kenya, Chicago, Brooklyn, or anywhere else, I realized in that room of starving and sick kids that I needed more than just a professional grasp of disease pathology. I needed a plan.

The children and adolescent room and the room with older kids were much easier for me to handle emotionally than the room with infants. Although the older kids were a little more self-sufficient, they were still sick and deeply vulnerable. Without treatment, many would be in dire straits. Yet despite their afflictions, some of them would run around, smiling and hopeful.

I always smiled back and waved when I saw the kids. My Swahili was limited to *habari yako*, which translates to "how are you?" The children giggled when I said it. I'm sure my accent was way off. Paul, one of the Kenyan medical students, said *habari yako* was a formal way of saying "how are you." "Children don't speak like that," he said. "Tell them *sassa* instead." "*Sassa*?" I asked uncertainly. "Yes, *sassa*. It's Sheng." Sheng is Swahili and English slang, a dialect spoken by young people in Kenya. *Sassa* means "speak," and the response to it is *fiit*, or "I'm cool." I hadn't heard of Sheng, but Paul and Njoroge, a new friend and Kenyan medical student, suggested I use that greeting instead, so I figured it was safe.

A few of the children approached me in the ward. Some came with curious stares like one three-year-old girl. She had the most beautiful and infectious smile. Even though she recently had her right eye removed because of a retinoblastoma tumor, she waved frantically and then ran away as to get me and the other students to engage her in her version of tag or hide-and-seek.

In Black culture, whether in the US, the Caribbean, or on the African continent, it is the unspoken words and gestures that are the most powerful, not just in acknowledging one another but in solidifying our bonds to one another. One day, three of the older children walked over to me and sized me up. They looked me over, from my feet to head and back down, as I was an unfamiliar face in their temporary home. The stares turned to smiles, and a few of the older children approached first and shook my hand in a way that was both identical to and acceptable across Black neighborhoods across the US and now apparently in Nairobi too. As a kid, I was taught the importance of a firm handshake. Black elders warned us of being judged based on our handshakes, suggesting that it needed to be done properly. Firm and standard for elders, creative for your peers, but never weak or limp. Our handshakes represented strength, power, and confidence. They gave a regional identification of where you were from or established an understanding between two people without verbal language.

The three boys were named Michael, Nicholas, and Vincent. I knew the names of these three because the nurses, other kids, medical students, and physicians regularly shouted at them. Nicholas and Vincent, both twelve years old, were both brilliant and natural comedians; both were being treated for Burkitt's lymphoma, a type of cancer that affects the lymph nodes. Nicholas had the oral form of Burkitt's, including a characteristic swelling of the face, making it difficult to chew or swallow. Vincent had the abdominal form of Burkitt's, which was a little more discreet. They had both been living in the hospital for some time, as they were being treated with chemotherapy on and off for the past three months. They were well acquainted with the hospital staff and KNH had become their home. Burkitt's lymphoma was always somehow a test question in medical school, but the likelihood of seeing it back home was scant. Nicholas spoke a little English and was very comfortable with greetings and salutations, but Vincent was completely fluent and became my official translator for the other children in the pediatric ward.

Then there was Michael. "*Sassa*," I spoke to him. "*Fiit*," he replied smiling back at me. "Hello, Michael," boomed a voice. "Hi, Michael," shouted another, until a series of hellos erupted around the room from the staff and medical students. Michael wasn't as talkative as Vincent, or as mischievous as Nicholas, but just as likable and friendly. He was eight years old, standing about three and a half feet tall, smiling and waddling while he walked. He didn't look sickly, aside from the minimal mucus crust around his nose like many of the other kids, and was just a little shorter than the other eight-year-olds. Maybe he had short parents. What was his story? "Why is he here?" I asked Njoroge, who replied, "He has AIDS, and he doesn't have anywhere else to go."

Kenya had an HIV/AIDS crisis with around three million infected in the country, many of whom didn't even know they were HIV positive. Much of sub-Saharan Africa had an HIV/AIDS crisis. Anywhere throughout the diaspora where Black and Brown people lived there seemed to be some kind of crisis. AIDS's looming presence just happened to be one of them. Reading reports about HIV/AIDS didn't do it justice because unless you lived there, knew someone dying of AIDS, or saw its impact as part of your work and school reality, there wasn't a real connection to the problem.

More than statistics, these were people. The numbers were mothers, fathers, sisters, brothers, and, in Michael's case, orphans.

Both of his parents had died from AIDS. Although Michael had AIDS he wasn't being treated for a particular illness that immunocompromised patients can commonly get. I'm still not even sure if he was taking antiretroviral medications, which are used to keep the HIV viral load down, dampen its impact on the body, and decrease the risk of transmission. Michael lived among the other patients his age on Ward 3D as an unofficial, permanent resident. The nurses on the ward took a liking to Michael and cared for him in the hospital. After he had first been treated in the hospital for an illness, there was no one to pick him up to take home. He had no family that would take him in and if he didn't stay in the hospital, he would be on the street.

"What about orphanages? Or extended family?" I asked Paul and Njoroge. "The families don't want them because of the stigma that they are connected to someone who has HIV. There aren't enough orphanages to take care of the kids, so they live on the street instead."

I felt my broken heart in my chest as I listened. A "damn" was all the response I could muster. I didn't know where to start or how to process this reality that existed for so many. Orphans living in the hospital. Patients sharing beds with even sicker patients. Parents and family sleeping on the floor. Some of the patients and their families came from all over the country to receive medical care at KNH and spent more money than they could afford just to travel to Nairobi. For them, the standard being provided at KNH was of higher quality than the small village clinics (that is, if there even was a clinic in their respective village). I was glad that KNH even existed. At least a modicum of care was being provided to the poor, but it wasn't enough.

There were a few issues taking place that impacted the care of the patients. The first was access. The doctors and nurses and other medical staff members regularly looked overworked. It didn't take a degree in rocket science to comprehend this. The World Health Organization (WHO) recommends 4.5 skilled health workers per 1,000 people. Africa and Southeast Asia, have the highest burdens of preventable diseases in the world and house some of the poorest regions in the world. They also have the lowest density of health workers per 1,000 people (2.2 in Africa and 3.3 in Southeast Asia). The Americas and Europe respectively have 9.6 and 14 skilled health workers per 1,000 people.[3]

KNH was obviously overcrowded, and putting patients in close proximity to one another increased the spread of communicable illnesses. It was also no different from any other public or government hospital in the developing world and resembled health care in certain parts of the US. Respiratory infections and diarrheal illnesses were, and still are, among the top five causes of death in Africa.[4] If there was more space to care for patients, I'm sure it would have been used.

In addition to the potential spread of infection in cramped quarters, it was cumbersome working in crowded wards. Overcrowding and limited hospital staff led to prolonged states of illness. It took longer for people to be cared for, and the longer they stayed, the sicker they got.

I wondered if it was unfair to judge the conditions based on a surface understanding of my new environment. I made assumptions after only a week in the country. Nonetheless, I still used a standard question: would I want to be treated there if I had another option? If I could afford to go to a private hospital with no crowding and beds with clean sheets, I would have gone, but that was an aspect of the problem. If one could avoid standards not to their liking and go elsewhere, they would. However, if no one advocated on behalf of those with limited options and brought in resources to improve the conditions that were substandard, how would the standards improve? That applies to neighborhoods and schools in the US and globally as well. It made me want to understand even more about improving the quality of health conditions.

In two months I was going to be a doctor, and the issues that impacted my future patients were going to be my problem. Even though I was going into emergency medicine to care for acute problems, I needed to think more about preventive health if I was to practice in resource-poor or resource-limited communities.

———————

I was done with studying for the day and caught up with Maureen and Winnie, also Kenyan medical students, and friends of my classmates from Buffalo who were at KNH a few months prior. They, too, had talked themselves out of studying and invited me to go with them to downtown Nairobi to check their email.

Most medical students didn't have computers, and there weren't phone lines set up in the dormitory rooms that allowed for an internet connection. For my new Kenyan friends, it was customary to travel to one of the various internet cafés littered around Nairobi to surf the internet, check email, or make long-distance phone calls. It was a little inconvenient to travel fifteen minutes to check email, but I kind of liked being able to disconnect from technology. Other than traveling on tightly packed buses devoid of personal space and the eight-hour time difference between Nairobi and New York City (I accidentally woke up my mother at 4 a.m. one day), it wasn't that bad. I looked at it as another way to explore unfamiliar territory beyond the confines of the medical school campus.

I managed to be close to the window of the crowded bus and had a chance to look at Nairobi's urban landscape. There were numerous tall, Western-style buildings and street merchants selling their goods, ranging from fruits to cookies and candies. Most of the people on the street were dressed and looked similar to those back home with the exception of a few Maasai. Some of the Maasai wore Western clothes but had characteristic elongated earlobes able to fit rounded disks as jewelry, as Maureen pointed out. Others wore more obvious leather sandals, colored necklaces and bracelets on their arms with long checkered shawls to cover their bodies in ways that their ancestors had been doing prior to the arrival of colonizers.

There were a number of teens walking down the street, coming from school, donning matching khaki shirt and pants or checkered short-sleeve shirts, likely to be their school uniforms. Just as there were groups of children in formalized uniforms, there were other children wearing a different type of uniform: dirty, tattered clothes, sometimes with flip-flops or barefoot. They were not in a formal school. They were called "street kids."

The street kids weren't hanging out after school and wearing beat-up play clothes so as to avoid tarnishing their uniforms. The street kids were homeless and orphaned. They were a small fraction of the more than one hundred thousand undomiciled youth in and around Nairobi and left to survive on their own.

"Why so many?" I asked Maureen. I really wanted to know why any at all, but that was a conversation that I didn't want to dive into as yet. "We think many of them were orphaned because their parents died from AIDS and there was no one to take them in," she said. "Many of the street kids might also be HIV positive." It made me think about Michael, the patient from pediatric ward 3D, who could have potentially been one of the kids if the nurses didn't keep him in the hospital.

Panhandling adults were a familiar sight to me in New York, but this was the first time I'd actually seen kids in such dire straits. Until I saw it firsthand, it felt too cruel to be real. Since I had arrived in Nairobi, I'd see an occasional "street kid," but today there they were, all together in multiple groups. Some were by themselves; others walked or sat together on the ground leaning against random walls and holding out their hands for money. Who were they? Where were their parents or other family members? Was this their family? I wondered about their individual stories of how they got there. I was curious how they survived but didn't really want to know so I didn't ask them. I really wished I could unsee what I saw. And that was the problem. I wanted to glamorize and romanticize Kenya, and the continent as a whole, or any other place I'd travel to as an exotic utopia, but it wasn't.

I was almost a doctor, and it was part of my plan to help alleviate suffering. Kenya felt different because I was unfamiliar with the reality, and it made me nervous. I felt like I should know how to address the issues I was seeing, but how do you address something if you've never been able to intimately connect with the problem? I didn't know how to address the poverty in front of me. Should I just share the children's stories with my friends? Should I give money? Adverse childhood experiences were ever present. Maybe if I gave money, that would make me a target for others to ask for money. Could I get robbed? Was it OK to speak to them and say "hello" or "*habari yako*" or "*sassa*"? Did I really want to know how they were doing or was it just a formality without genuine concern?

There was a group of street kids sitting on the sidewalk and asking for money. This was a much larger group than the others as there were about six or maybe eight of them. They ranged in age from about two or three years old to about fourteen, with the eldest being a girl with shortly cropped hair and a long dark-green shirt dress. She kept the kids in line, organizing, consoling, disciplining, and looking after them as their mother. I had no way of knowing if she was biologically related to the others. She could have been the oldest sister or just someone who decided to look after the others and created her own community to improve their chances of surviving.

Minnie suggested we could give them milk since there was a supermarket down the block. We purchased a few personalized containers of milk from the Nakumat supermarket and gave the containers to the young matriarch donning the green dress. She smiled and said "*asante sana*," the Swahili phrase for "thank you very much," and proceeded to evenly distribute the milk to her group. I have never been able to forget that scene, and I hope I never will. It serves as a constant reminder to me of the ravages of poverty globally, and how much work we all need to do to begin to address it.

I learned in my time in Kenya, as do so many others who visit parts of the world so much more disadvantaged than their own, that economic injustice and the poverty bred of colonialism cause cycles of terrible violence that seep into the fabric of societies. They create not just discomfort but lifelong consequences and illnesses that threaten the basis of human existence. The people suffering and dying from curable medical illnesses are the same who suffer from acts of violence. There is no separation. This kind of systemic injustice is very much parallel to what happens in societies everywhere, including all over the US. To ignore the injustices is to accept that some life is unworthy, particularly the lives of those who look like me. The question of how this continued to happen stood like a heavy shadow behind every patient I cared for in Kenya. And the answers to that question couldn't easily be compartmentalized; nor should they be. In order to move beyond accepting that certain groups were destined to have shorter lives filled with deprivation, I needed to do more and understand more.

CHAPTER 8

SOMETHING EXCITING

IT WAS AUGUST IN CHICAGO, usually a scorcher, in the nineties to low hundreds. My apartment was hot and I was running low on popsicles. The air conditioner in Clifford, my big red Chevy Cavalier, was out of commission. I had what my grandfather called "the people's air," aka rolling down the window and praying for a breeze. The hottest days of the summer usually saw the most victims of violence, likely because unrelenting heat made people uncomfortable and irritable and everyone who stayed outside hoping for a breeze got more agitated in that discomfort. But this particular day was different. It was in the fifties and rainy, a welcome change. I was on call, and the trauma emergency department at Cook County Hospital was going to be my home for the next twenty-four hours. I hoped for a quiet shift.

That day the trauma ED was unbelievably quiet, a rare state. There's a superstition in emergency departments that you never talk about how quiet it is. We all believe that the minute anyone says that, the patients will flood in as if from a breached dam. I was chief resident by then and had a shitload of other work to do even on a quiet day. My red, black, and green bookbag was a vessel for self-replicating paperwork, and I could really have used a few extra hours devoid of patients to catch up on some of it.

Even though that was true, as much as we claimed to long for quiet, motion, activity, and adrenaline rushes were often welcomed for us in emergency medicine. This was 2005, there were no smartphones packed with distractions to pass the time—we just had each other and surfed the internet, doing random Google and Yahoo searches on things that came to mind. I had my paperwork but not everyone had even that. After puttering around awhile, one of our team members said, "I'm bored." Sure enough, group mentality prevailed, and immediately most of my colleagues chimed in, agreeing with a "Yeah," almost in unison. He then continued with, "I hope something exciting comes in!" Herd mentality continued with another chorus of "Yeah, we need something exciting to come in!"

"Something exciting" meant one thing: trauma. Specifically, penetrating trauma coming in the form of a gunshot or stab wound. Resident physicians preferred to have patients coming in with penetrating trauma rather than blunt trauma. With blunt trauma, the injury is the result of impact from a surface or firm object that doesn't penetrate the skin. Blunt trauma can be caused by fists, furniture, and other objects, and the injuries range from bumps and bruises to death caused by a fall or a car accident, but the workups of those patients were long and arduous, consisting of multiple X-rays taken by Fred, our hardworking and good-natured, but not-all-that-skilled, X-ray tech. Fred's work often had to be done over, making dealing with blunt trauma even more frustrating.

Penetrating trauma meant there were opportunities for us to perform trauma resuscitation surgical procedures—there's a reason that there are so many of them on medical TV shows. Treating penetrating trauma is dramatic and fast, and requires intense concentration and focus. You might have to intubate someone, placing a 7.5 mm plastic tube into their throat to help them breathe. Or you might have to do a complex laceration repair on the face. There was a specific kind of wound we saw regularly that we called a "buck fifty" or a "smiley face." The buck fifty came from the fact that a very large laceration could take as many as 150 sutures or more to repair. It left a scar that was called the "smiley face" because it went from the side of the cheek across to the victim's mouth, almost mimicking the smile of the Joker in Batman movies.

I'd been told that this type of injury, usually caused by a knife, razor, or broken bottle, was done for the sole purpose of humiliating the victim. Scars on the belly or chest could be hidden by clothes but hiding disfiguring scars on the face is impossible.

Other procedures common in patients with penetrating trauma included tubes to assist in draining air or blood, or sometimes both, from the chest after something sharp had pierced it. A cricothyrotomy, or "cric," involved using a scalpel to slice a tiny hole in a very precise spot in the neck to help a patient breathe in the event of massive swelling that could cause the patient's airway to collapse. I had only ever done this on a cadaver. Probably the most coveted procedure was "cracking the chest," also known as a thoracotomy, a potentially lifesaving procedure that involved opening up the chest with a scalpel to see the organs of the thoracic cavity. With a thoracotomy, the team would be able to perform a number of other procedures like draining blood from around the heart in the case of cardiac tamponade, massaging the heart, or clamping down on injured blood vessels to prevent the patient from bleeding to death by diverting blood to vital organs like the heart and the brain. It took skill, focus, precision, and was the bloodiest procedure imaginable. Those who did them, whether successfully saving a life or not, wore a badge of honor.

As one of the few resident physicians who had had the opportunity to assist with opening up someone's chest after the patient had been shot, I had not only this feeling of power, because I had developed and used skills to save someone's life, but a sense of pride, because I would be able to share war stories with friends and colleagues who weren't in that elite club. We all wanted to have those stories, almost as an induction into a special brother- or sisterhood. When an elder emergency doc or trauma surgeon shared their stories of working on "the front lines" in the medical trenches of urban warfare of the 1980s and '90s crack wars, they took on a legendary status for us rookies. They were heroes in our eyes, and we wanted to be heroes with better and more exciting stories. The thrill we sought was both biological and psychological. A rush of endogenous norepinephrine is released at our synaptic clefts during high-stress experiences. These chemicals provide a unique type of euphoria, similar to being high, which makes it easy to get caught up in the excitement of our work—and sometimes forget what is really happening to the person, so often a young man, we are working on.

For some reason, this day hit me differently. What we were calling "exciting" meant that most likely another Black or Latino male in his teens or twenties would be brought in, gravely injured in the type of battle that never has a victor. The patient that my colleagues dubbed "exciting" looked like me or one of my friends or cousins. Most likely, their families came up to the northern parts of the US from the Deep South like Alabama, Mississippi, or Georgia—like my family—or from Mexico and settled in Chicago for better opportunities. But the inconsistent dolling of opportunities by the hands of fate brought us together in the ED.

I felt like a hypocrite. I wanted to do procedures and check off boxes and tell stories like the seasoned veteran docs, but to satisfy my professional desires we needed a constant supply of bodies. At Cook County, they were all too often Black or Brown bodies.

I looked around the room. I was the only Black physician there. The only other person in the room was the clerk. I began to feel even more conflicted and uneasy. It was a paradox. We all—including me—needed the training and real-world skill development that working in a busy urban ED provided. I particularly wanted to develop these skills because I wanted to keep working in a city ED, preferably back in Brooklyn. If I didn't learn how to work well under pressure, people could lose their lives. So in that way, having to work on these traumatic injuries was a terrible necessity.

But as we referred to the people who had received these injuries as "exciting," as though their suffering was there for our amusement, I began to feel like I was taking part in a sort of experiment on the people who were our patients. Not that we weren't doing good, trying to keep people alive—but that we were contributing to a system that kept the trauma going.

Many of the doctors who came to Cook County for their residency training went on to work at what were referred to as "real world" institutions. What that phrase often meant was going to work at a private hospital with tons of resources.

That term "real world" began to make me angry. Was Cook County Hospital not a real place? Were the patients there, mostly Black and poor, not also real people with real problems? Cook County Hospital had been in Chicago since 1847, serving mostly the Black population—in the 1960s, 80 percent of the city's Black births and 50 percent of Black deaths took place there.[1] While there was no official, legal segregation, by virtue of custom, location, and, ultimately, bias, it was *the* Black hospital. My father was born at Cook County Hospital. My grandmother had all but one of her children there. For me, it wasn't just another "killer county," a casually cruel nickname thrown around in reference to many of the public hospitals across the US.

But was I another young doctor there to experiment? Did the patients we treated feel like they were being experimented on? I felt guilty for wanting to see trauma. Maybe I felt like this because what was being done was a Band-Aid approach to a larger issue, one that wasn't being addressed at the systemic level. I started to be convinced that I had to do something more than stitching up victims . . . but what?

Grand rounds is an old tradition in academic medical centers where topics related to patient pathology or trauma are presented. Doing grand rounds as resident physician is a chance to present before your peers, supervising physicians and surgeons, students, and the entire department and comment on a major trend or issue in medicine. Every resident has to present at grand rounds, and some welcome it while others just want to get it out of the way. Either way, there was usually something to be learned from the person doing the presentation, offering new and interesting ideas on health and ways to treat disease. I had already made a number of presentations at Cook about specific core topics in emergency medicine: Kawasaki disease, testicular torsion, clonidine overdoses, trauma in pregnancy, and genitourinary trauma. But I hadn't done grand rounds yet.

My grand rounds presentation was to be in February, a time of year in Chicago when the negative-degree cold made a walk to the car feel like a polar expedition. Inspired by the weather, I was looking forward to presenting on hypothermia, but another resident called dibs. I was left trying to figure out what to do next.

I met with my program director and faculty advisor, Dr. Steve Bowman and he urged me to present on something with a larger societal impact. He suggested I take a look at a book he just finished reading called *Freakonomics*, by University of Chicago faculty members Steven D. Levitt and Stephen J. Dubner.[2] The book posits that there's a hidden economic basis to everything that we do. I read the book immediately.

One of the book chapters was titled "Why Do Drug Dealers Still Live with Their Moms?" The chapter described how Sudhir Venkatesh, a grad student from India studying sociology, spent time with the Black Gangster Disciples (sometimes referred to as Black Disciples, Gangster Disciples, or GD), a well-known Chicago gang on the South Side that functioned with a militaristic type of organizational structure. Venkatesh spent several years with the members, visiting their families, and sometimes even sleeping in their apartments. His research, as well as the chapter in the book by Levitt and Dubner, directly addressed poverty in the Black community, how the gang began dealing crack cocaine, how they worked to create its economic infrastructure, and how they collectively assessed risk and conducted cost-benefit analysis. This mode of thinking helped me begin to crystallize some thoughts about what I'd been observing in the ED as it related specifically to violence.

During my residency, I'd seen more grievous violence-related injuries than I could even remember. And almost always there was a clear pattern:

1. Patients come to the hospital with injuries caused at the hands of another—sometimes fatal, sometimes not.
2. The survivors are often taken to the operating room to be patched up.
3. Superficial injuries are treated in the emergency department and the patients are discharged home with pain medication.

4. Discharged patients are told to "be careful" and to come back to the trauma clinic for follow-up appointments.

5. Often, patients didn't come in for the follow-up appointments. But over and over we did see them return with new violence-caused injuries. Or someone else would come in with an injury caused by a former patient. Far more than I cared to think about, patients—especially young men—came back reinjured and reinjured again until they finally came back to be pronounced dead.

One of my earliest cases that followed this pattern was typical: KC, as he was called, was twenty-four. He was an OG, an "Original Gangsta," a title given to the "baddest mothafuckers" that younger gangbangers looked up to, the ones who called the shots.

He had a fresh haircut faded on the sides and a neatly trimmed goatee consisting of only a beard and mustache—probably because he wasn't old enough for his beard to connect to his mustache. He was close to six foot two inches tall, with a muscular build and a few tattoos on his biceps. None of it seemed to matter, because he was dead.

When you've been shot, or stabbed in the chest, there are several different things that can kill you. The pleural membrane, which is the membrane surrounding the lung, can be pierced, causing air and blood to rush in and fill the chest cavity, collapsing the lung and preventing you from breathing. The bullet, or any sharp object (such as a knife), can hit the esophagus, trachea, heart, lung tissue itself, the great vessels of the heart, and other major blood vessels, depending on the angle.

In some cases, we try the thoracotomy; by then I had seen a few of those. But it was too late for KC—by the time he arrived he was what we called at County a "triple zero"—not breathing, no blood pressure, and no heart rate. The thoracotomy was unsuccessful and KC was pronounced dead shortly after. Another brotha gone before his prime. It hurt to see this—once again he could have been me or someone from my neighborhood.

According to the Chicago Police Department, KC was a drug dealer but also had a reputation for killing people, an assassin of sorts. We closed the gaping hole in his chest wall prior to his family viewing the body because it would have been an even larger emotional burden if the family saw what he looked like before we sewed him up. The blood that ran down his arms and chest had stained his palms, so he looked like the saddened Jesus statues that adorned the walls of my Catholic high school. His friends and family mourned and wailed at their loss. I don't think they were oblivious to his past as a gangbanger and an OG, but still they cried. Maybe they mourned because of innocence that had been lost, remembering him as a child who played with his friends before he got caught up in street life.

The nurses and ER techs wrapped up his body in white sheets to make it as presentable as possible to the distraught family members coming in. KC kind of looked like the funeral pictures of Malcolm X (el-Hajj Malik el-Shabazz) I studied as a teen. KC was dead and covered in white, but his face wasn't turned east to Mecca like Malcolm X in his funeral garb after his untimely passing, and people didn't refer to KC as our "Shining Black Prince." I didn't know KC's story. I didn't cry. I had been employed at Cook County for less than a year and a half and this had already become routine in my work, almost as regular an occurrence as someone catching a cold.

There were many others like KC who came in, and the scenarios all mirrored each other. Like the many different teenagers who arrived shot after school, the twenty-something-year-olds sprayed up after leaving the club, the bottle strikes to the head and the stab wounds to the chest after guys had a night out of drinking, the guys who were shot execution style in a warehouse just minutes away from the hospital.

I'll never forget the faces of the families that came in to mourn the dead. Their slow walks down the hall to the empty room where the body is kept before taking it to the morgue. The screams from the mothers. The way their sisters fell to the ground. The self-blaming of the brothers. The regrets of the uncles. The talk of revenge. The promise that more bodies would be landing in the emergency department. I knew there would be more bodies to come because that was what always happened, like clockwork. Someone got shot and then another person got shot who was somehow connected to the initial person who got shot, and the family and neighborhood were left to deal with the repercussions. It was a vicious cycle of violence with no beneficiaries other than the companies that manufactured the weapons, and maybe the ones that made the coffins. His was the kind of story I wanted to tell. This would become the subject of my grand rounds.

In preparing for my grand rounds presentation, I threw myself into understanding the root causes of violence and into work around violence prevention, reading everything I could get my hands on. I came across the work of Dr. John Rich, who is now the inaugural director of the Rush BMO Institute for Health Equity at the Rush University System of Health in Chicago. Dr. Rich wrote a paper titled "Pathways to Recurrent Trauma Among Young Black Men: Traumatic Stress, Substance Use, and the 'Code of the Street.'"[3]

Reading his paper and his interviews was the first time I ever read someone describe violence as a public health problem, where you have these risk factors that are identifiable, just like any other disease process. If you mitigate the impact of those different risk factors, you can potentially change the outcome for the people and populations being impacted. I started thinking if a person who had experienced violence had had an intervention earlier on, this entire person's life trajectory could be completely different. I started reading more of Dr. Rich's work and the work of Dr. Arthur Kellerman, an emergency physician and early pioneer in gun violence prevention; I was like a mad person. I started identifying other people who had done these interventions and read more about their work and started meeting with them. As I did my research on gun violence and gang violence, I realized that at the time—in 2005 and 2006—there weren't many intervention programs out there. I went wild trying to find out what were the best ways to implement these types of programs.

One of the programs I came across was called Caught in the Crossfire from the Oakland, California, nonprofit called Youth ALIVE! The first hospital-based violence intervention program in the country, Youth ALIVE! was working with Highland Hospital, an exceptionally busy public hospital in a predominantly Black neighborhood and directly tied to the community it was part of in a particular and unusual way. It was started by Sherman Spears, a young man who described himself in a 1998 interview as "a high-profile violent type of person."[4] He was shot and paralyzed and came to the conclusion that there had to be a way out this cycle of violence. The only support he received from friends and family after he was shot was encouragement to take revenge—he came to believe that there was another way of reconciling with violence. Bit by bit, the way developed.

Caught in the Crossfire was shaped around the idea that if immediate support could be provided directly to victims of violence in the hospitals, it would help prevent retaliatory violence and give the patients and their families the support needed. The current mission statement of Youth ALIVE!, the nonprofit that manages Caught in the Crossfire, spells it out. This is from the 2022 website but the mission has always been the same:

> Since 1991, as mentors, youth leaders, counselors, case managers, intervention specialists and violence interrupters, we at Youth ALIVE! have worked to help violently wounded people heal themselves and their community. Our mission is to prevent violence and create young leaders. We believe that young people growing up and going to school in the city's most violent neighborhoods possess the power to change the city for the better. We meet our clients where they are, at home, in school, at the hospital bedsides of young shooting victims, on the streets of our most dangerous neighborhoods.
>
> Our frontline staff is composed of men and women who grew up in the communities they serve. Some are former victims, some former gang members. All are highly trained in the best practices of their profession. They bring not judgement, but only understanding, knowledge, and a path to greater peace for traumatized individuals and the city.

Our primary goals along the way to achieving our mission are these:

1. To educate and train young leaders to create a more peaceful community
2. To interrupt the cycle of violence on the streets
3. To convince angry victims and their loved ones not to retaliate
4. To provide ongoing support to help the wounded and grieving get needed services and heal from their trauma.[5]

An approach like this was the one I'd been searching for. As my research continued I found out that my mentor, Dr. Thea James, had developed another hospital-based violence intervention program, the Violence Intervention and Advocacy Program, based at Boston Medical Center (BMC), then called Boston City Hospital. Learning this was like being a miner, unearthing veins of gold ore spreading across the country, a rich and beautiful discovery.

Public health is defined as "the science and art of preventing disease, prolonging life and promoting health through the organized efforts and informed choices of society, organizations, public and private, communities and individuals."[6] In order for a disease to occur, a person has to be exposed to a pathogen. The type of pathogen, how rapidly it multiplies, and the strength of a person's immune system will determine if the person will develop symptoms of that disease. The type of stressors a person routinely deals with and how frequently they are exposed to a disease will partially determine if they will have a recurrence of that disease.

It made complete sense. Violent injuries were recurrent based on my own observations, the experiences of my patients, and as documented in scientific journals. Violence proliferated just like an infectious disease.

Highland Hospital in Oakland and BMC were very much like Cook County Hospital, where I worked, and similar to Kings County Hospital back in Brooklyn. The major difference was that something was being done at those hospitals beyond patching people up and hoping for the best.

I was nervous before my presentation but also fired up to share my new thinking and all that I'd learned. The impassive faces of the senior doctors gazed at me as I put up my first slide.

There had been 5,570 homicides in the United States in 2003. The country's firearm homicide rate was seventeen times higher than that of other industrialized nations, and homicide was the number-two cause of death for US youth that year. Of those more than five thousand homicides, most victims were Black.[7]

I talked about how often we, as emergency physicians, see recurrent victims and how I'd been learning that the "code of the street," as explicated in Elijah Anderson's book with that title, meant that a victim of violence who did not respond aggressively to an attack was, in essence, tolerating victimization.[8]

I talked about John Rich's theory of "pathways to recurrence"— the ways in which ACEs, the code of the street, trauma and lack of faith in the police led to recurrence. I then outlined what was beginning to become my vision.

Drawing on the work of Dr. Kurt Denninghoff, I pointed out that we, as emergency docs, failed our patients who had been victims (or even perpetrators) of violence by not being prepared to conduct interventions, not having the resources to refer patients to help that might break the cycle, not having established intervention protocols but instead focusing only on the consequences of violence—patching people up and sending them back out the door.[9] As the first to encounter victims of violence, we could be the front line in changing the response if we developed the resources. My thoughts were nascent at that time—I suggested something as simple as perhaps passing out a brochure about community resources. A Band-Aid on a gaping wound. But it was the beginning of my journey into a new way of thinking.

CHAPTER 9

THE PIPELINE

WHEN I FIRST EXPRESSED interest in being a doctor, I had a couple of lucky breaks, breaks that people of color who are interested in medicine don't always get. The first happened when I was just seventeen, still running cross-country in high school, and came in the form of a mentor. My mother had an orthopedic problem and one of her teaching colleagues recommended a Dr. Answorth Allen. The woman ranted about how smart, friendly, and skilled Dr. Allen was and gave him the thumbs-up. Naturally, my mother felt comfortable going to see the surgeon, given this high recommendation. Wanting to have a great surgeon was important; however, my mother was pleasantly surprised after walking in to see Dr. Allen that he was Black. My mother's colleague was an Orthodox Jewish woman, so to be honest, along with our own biases and limitations in visual representation with doctors, we hadn't thought about her surgeon being a Black man. My mother came back home after her evaluation and couldn't wait to tell me that her new doctor was a young Black guy, only in his early thirties.

"I told him all about you, that you wanted to be a doctor. He's even a sports doctor," she said. I was excited and couldn't wait to meet him. I also needed to see him as a patient. I had a new knee injury, likely from overtraining (I ran five hundred miles that summer training for cross-country), so I needed an appointment to see Dr. Allen before my cross-country season started in a few weeks.

Dr. Allen looked nothing what I perceived doctors to look like or act like. He hailed from Jamaica, West Indies, but had been in the US for some time. He shook my hand and seemed genuinely happy to meet me. He didn't even have to say much because I was in awe. Dots in my head started connecting ideas and thoughts about working in a space like this and treating people for medical problems. We spoke initially about school and what he did as an orthopedic surgeon and about sports and athletic performance and how the human body handles it. It was a brilliant way to transition into focusing on my issues as a patient and almost made me forget about my ailment. Dr. Allen examined me and—after a series of questions and twists, torques, and pressing on my knee—told me I had plica syndrome, a condition involving the tissue in my knee joint that caused clicking and pain, typically due to an injury or overuse. The prescription was rest, something I wasn't a fan of. More thrilling than the good prognosis he gave me about my knee was the conversation we had about my hopes of becoming a doctor. He said, in so many words, "If you want to be a doc, we'll get you there."

Shortly after that visit, he let me, a kid in high school, shadow him in the hospital, his clinic, and in the operating room. He gave me scrubs to wear, taught me how to scrub in to surgery, and allowed me to watch him repair a meniscal tear and do ACL reconstructive surgery. I stood next to him during the procedures, and he even let me suction blood from an area of the patient that was bleeding. In retrospect, the task was pretty minimal, but back then I felt like I was operating. I learned other stuff from him too, like how to do a knee examination to check for function, stability, and injuries. He and one of his colleagues took me out to eat at a fancy restaurant on the Upper East Side—I had to look halfway decent and learn how to use all the appropriate silverware. That restaurant experience would teach me some valuable lessons that I would call on later, like how to navigate through philanthropic spaces and fundraisers, raising money and meeting donors. I really appreciated that teaching.

Besides the operating room experience, a few years later when I was in college, Dr. Allen hired me to work in his office, doing paperwork, filing, and other administrative tasks. It was boring sometimes but that, too, is part of the life of a doctor, and it was good to be exposed to it. I also joined him when he had clinic and occasionally went to the operating room when he had cases. He was a really special guy and is still an important figure to me.

According to the 2015 Association of American Medical Colleges report *Altering the Course: Black Males in Medicine*: "In 1978 there were 542 Black male matriculants to medical school and in 2014 we had 515."[1] The number of Black men in medicine had decreased, but the Black population hadn't. When I was a young man with very high ambitions, having Black role models was key to my confidence and progress, and now, years later, I recognize that I need to pay that forward and be a mentor myself. Not all BIPOC professionals are comfortable in such a role, and some even express resentment about it, feeling it's someone else's responsibility. I get that, but I also understand the unquestionable value of a role model, and I, for one, recognize that representation matters, and so I willingly mentor, happy to be a role model whenever I can be.

In 2006, when I returned to Brooklyn after completing my residency at Cook County Hospital, I began working at Kings County Hospital and SUNY Downstate Medical Center, the fraternal twins of medical care in East Flatbush. Kings was run by the city, and SUNY was run by the state. They sit across the street from one another, with Kings County also across the street from my elementary school. At that point, I was completely launched on my mission about addressing violence as a public health issue. I'd done a fair amount of study and research since my grand rounds presentation back in Chicago. And now that I was home, I had an ally in Dr. Ray Austin, the first Black male emergency medicine doctor I'd ever met, back in 2001, when I did an away rotation as a visiting medical student through Kings County Hospital. Dr. Austin shared my passion for addressing violence systemically and had been part of starting a small group called Doctors Against Murder.

DAM had big aspirations, but by the time I returned to Brooklyn, it was pretty much defunct, hobbled by a lack of funds and by the fact that everyone involved was a busy practicing physician. No one had time to devote to what it took to get an anti-violence program going. Dr. Austin and I didn't give up though. We talked often, snatching time while on shift and meeting before or after work, shaping our ideas.

We kept talking and then gradually, I started working on proposals, writing, and rewriting them and beginning to believe that building the program was possible. Whenever an opportunity came up to discuss youth violence or gun violence at a conference or even in the hospital, I jumped at it. These smaller, intimate conversations morphed into other opportunities to speak with larger groups that shared my desire to understand and prevent community violence. I never hesitated to bring up the need for our hospital to have an intervention program and the need for financial support. Like clockwork, it was always the same boilerplate reply: "Wow, this is a great idea. But sorry, we don't have any money." Always, I'd push back, saying this could save the hospital money and keep people alive, but the response was always the same: a squeamish, twisted face saying how sorry they were.

It took many, many deep breaths, but after a while I acknowledged to myself that every presentation was another opportunity to tweak my sales pitch. I continued speaking at a series of different medical conferences in front of various groups, including nurses, hospital administrators, physicians and surgeons, educators, high school and middle school students, public health students and practitioners, concerned citizens, parents, and elected officials.

Back in 2006, the hospital had agreed to set up a meeting between state senator Eric Adams (who would be elected mayor of New York City in 2021), Dr. Austin, and myself, but nothing ever happened. Dr. Austin and I decided we could either continue to wait or do something. We decided to cold-call the senator and invite him to the hospital ourselves. In 2007, our perseverance paid off.

In a small conference room in the hospital the three of us spoke about a range of topics: the scope of violence, the need for intervention programs, the cost of financing such programs, and partnering with elected officials to influence policy. I felt great coming out of our conversation with Senator Adams. It was our first time talking to someone who might have access to the resources that it would take to make the program go. But the excitement wasn't shared everywhere. Hospital administrators were pissed about us meeting with the senator without their knowledge, even though they had been promising and failing to set up the meeting for a year. I didn't know we were supposed to let the higher-ups know in advance. But I didn't sweat it. The meeting didn't result in funding, but it was even more practice in engaging with elected officials and pitching ideas in the future. And I'd learned that asking for forgiveness rather than for permission was often the way to get things done.

In 2007, I became an assistant residency director for Kings County–SUNY Downstate's Department of Emergency Medicine. At the time, the residency program was one of the nation's largest; it is now the largest EM residency training program in the US. Residency directors, or program directors, are responsible for co-ordinating the teaching and training of new doctors in their given specialty. They are responsible for developing curriculums, management, and recruitment, to name a few tasks.

When I first started as an assistant residency director, I was the only "minority" on the team (that was the prevalent terminology at that time). One of the main reasons I wanted to be a residency director was because we didn't have any Black, Latino, or any other persons of color on the team. For a residency program based in East Flatbush, Brooklyn, which served two hospitals where more than 80 percent of the patient population identified as Black or of African descent, our program needed to be the Blackest and most colorful thing in existence.

There are numerous studies showing that physicians of color are important for all communities but especially for those where the doctors will be the same race as most of their patients. This line from a summation of a 2001 symposium on the need to diversify the health professions said it well: "Strong, compelling evidence suggests that minority physicians are indeed more likely to provide precisely those services that may be most likely to reduce racial and ethnic health disparities, namely primary care services for underserved poor and minority populations."[2] The authors go on to make a point that this doesn't mean that "minority physicians are being trained solely to provide health-care services to minority patients or to research minority health issues" but that a broader range of physicians would benefit all patients. What they said based on empirical evidence, I felt on a gut level every day.

When I was in medical school and in residency, I mentored medical students and premedical students of color. I spoke to them about getting into school or residency. I had them shadow me, just as doctors had allowed me to shadow them when I was younger. I knew what a difference it had made to me and I'm sure it mattered even more to them. But I knew we needed to do much more in order to truly build a pipeline of emergency doctors of color.

In 2009, I kind of snapped. It just came out. I usually slept like a log, no matter what happened on shift. But one night after a shift I couldn't sleep. Earlier in the day my boss, the residency director, Dr. Chris Doty, asked me why we weren't able to recruit many Black or Latino medical students into the residency that year. That question bugged me because I didn't have an answer. We had a pretty intense and well-intended interview season of recruiting top talent from around the world. We tried to recruit students of color, but we managed to have only a few match into our residency program. It kept bugging me that night and I thought, *We have got to find a way to increase the number of Black and Latinos in emergency medicine.* And that was it. Sleep was over for that night. I sat up writing a long email—and I don't write long emails—to Dr. Doty.

In the email I said that doctors of color don't come because we're not investing in them early enough. We reach out and maybe take them out to dinner when they're already fourth-year medical students. We've got to reach out and build relationships with them much earlier. The other problem: we were reaching out to the students that everyone was fighting for, the top 10 percent. I reasoned that we could be there to support students of color who were in the other 90 percent—not being at the top academically didn't mean they wouldn't be fine doctors. Doing great in school isn't a firm indicator of how a physician will behave at someone's bedside or of what's in their heart. And we could offer the mentoring they needed to become the best docs they could be.

Dr. Doty replied, "Rob, you've hit on something here. Let's take this further." Over the next few days, my email expanded into a detailed proposal that I would present to the steering committee of our Department of Emergency Medicine. I was so excited that I agreed to meet with them one late morning after being up all night from working the overnight shift in the emergency department. Sleep is always precious to both young and old docs, or anyone working in places of high stress, chaos, and organized confusion. I figured I would sleep when I was done with presenting; I felt that something greater was at stake. Sleep deprived but full of adrenaline, I knocked the presentation out. I knew I connected the thoughts and ideas with the steering committee by looking at how some of the senior docs adjusted the seating positions in their chairs. At the conclusion of my presentation the committee said they would get me the funding for this idea I had.

Over the next two to three months a program called Minority Medical Student Emergency Medicine (MMSEM) was born. Since 2009, we've nurtured more than a hundred medical students and premedical students of color through the program, most of whom go into the field of emergency medicine. Here it is, in a nutshell, from our application:

> MMSEM is designed to give highly qualified first and second year medical students the opportunity to get first-hand clinical experience in one of the busiest emergency departments in the country. In an intense 40 hour a week, 6-week program, participants will gain direct experience in emergency medicine research, clinical skills such as history taking, suturing, splinting, exposure to cutting edge emergency ultrasound and medical simulation, grant writing, USMLE [United States Medical Licensing Examination] and residency application preparation, and mentoring experience with the most diverse emergency medicine residency program in the country.

I'm proud that Kings County and SUNY Downstate help send emergency medicine docs of color all over the country and in other parts of the world. Having the docs of color in emergency departments builds trust, empathy, and compassion in these settings, which are so often filled with confusion, unease, and suspicion. What's more, doctors of color serve as role models, which is so crucial to building confidence for BIPOC community members.

My interest in trauma was still strong, and now I had the hands to work to develop hard data to support that interest. Students Ernesto Romo and Justin Britton (both emergency medicine physicians now) researched how to develop and enhance a comprehensive trauma registry that would expand the data our hospital was already collecting. Tolu Olade, another student (also now an emergency medicine physician), conducted research about violence prevention programs nationwide. There were sticky notes everywhere. These students were working sixty to eighty hours a week. It paid off. Three other student interns—Adrianne Stevenson (now an ob-gyn doctor), Sarah Jamison (now an emergency medicine doctor), and Michelle Garrido (now a family medicine doctor)—were tasked specifically with helping me develop a violence intervention program. At program's end, the students presented the fruits of their labor. Together they came up with the name KAVI, an acronym for Kings Against Violence Initiative. They proposed "Kings" not only as the name of the borough we were in (Brooklyn is also known as Kings County) but also because "Kavi" is Sanskrit for enlightened, poet, thinker, and doer. With KAVI, we hoped to shine a little light on this massive issue. Now to find a way to make it a reality.

CHAPTER 10

VIOLENCE IN THE RUBBLE

HISTORICALLY, I've always been accustomed to sleeping in places that others would call disagreeable: floors, benches, dentist chairs (a skill Moms and I share), and even inside noisy MRI machines. But this night I couldn't get settled to sleep and was up and down, periodically unnerved by things I noticed in the room around me in my new environment. The air was hot and muggy, and the single hole in my mosquito net threw me to the edge of paranoia, haunting me with the thought of a buzzing visitor who might give me malaria.

I'd always been sensitive to smells, both pleasant and unpleasant. The good smells of breakfast coming from a kitchen trigger pleasant memories. But the smell this morning was different: abrupt and unsettling. I'd smelled it before, passing an overturned car that had collided with a tractor-trailer on the highway. It was the same smell that wafted from firefighters who had recently put out a blaze, wearing the reminder of their latest work encounter. It was the smell of burning. Burning rubber, burning wood, burning plastic with its characteristic black smoke, and it reminded me of death.

There was indistinct chattering on the other side of my bedroom door. Something about problems with driving down the street and leaving the compound.

A few minutes after waking to the smell, our driver came in and said that my colleagues and I should expect delays in heading to the airport because there was a protest outside.

There was the threat of missing or being late for my emergency department shift the next day, but I cared less about missing my flight. I was more nervous about what was going on outside and whether it would come inside the walls. I couldn't even be mad. Travel delays and protests were to be expected. Burning car tires and demonstrations were almost universal signs of election protests in underdeveloped countries. Anything could happen; this was Haiti.

Because I grew up in central Brooklyn, which has the second-largest Haitian community in the US (second only to Miami), I'd felt connected to Haiti since I was very young. One of my favorite comic books from the Golden Legacy series was on Toussaint L'Ouverture. L'Ouverture was a Haitian general who helped lead his country's revolt against the French, resulting in Haiti being the first Black country to gain its independence from European colonial rule (Ethiopia is the only Black country never colonized). I liked the idea that the underdog overthrew an empire. Haiti's successful rebellion led to countless other rebellions around the world against European powers. I was impressed by L'Ouverture. He was a warrior and an educated intellectual, with an ability to bring people together. What wasn't to like about him and his story?

This was my seventh trip to Haiti, and it was two days after the one-year anniversary of the January 12, 2010, earthquake (I would eventually make a total of fourteen or fifteen trips to the beloved country). The shifting tectonic plates had unsettled many homes, businesses, and natural habitats, and disrupted the flow of people, water, resources, and almost all day-to-day activities. The earthquake cast new light on what the Haitian people already knew well: their country was poor, more people lived in poverty than didn't, and most didn't have reliable access to food, clean water, or basic medical care.

I was joined by my friend and colleague in the Department of Emergency Medicine Dr. Christina Bloem, the president of EMEDEX International, a nongovernmental organization (NGO) dedicated to the global expansion of emergency medicine and disaster preparedness. We would join local Haitian nurses and doctors from the Hopital Bernard Mevs, a private hospital in Port-au-Prince; trauma surgeons from the University of Miami; and staff from another NGO called Project Medishare to discuss developing an emergency medicine training program in the country's largest and busiest city.

From our previous trips to Haiti, Dr. Bloem, other team members, and I had learned a few things after setting up training programs with local medical professionals and educators:

1. Relationships take time to build.
2. Community stakeholders are valuable allies.
3. It's important to ask the stakeholders about the needs of the community, rather than making assumptions.
4. Having an in-depth understanding of the community is essential.
5. When nonlocal medics leave, the community should have the capacity to carry on in a sustainable way and improve what was built.

These insights would later become crucial in how KAVI was developed.

This current trip would serve twin purposes: our US team would be able to learn about the Haitian medical system and tropical medicine—which would be useful since a large number of patients in Brooklyn were from Haiti and other countries in the Caribbean—and, in turn, our team would share our medical insights while helping train local laborers, drivers, medical professionals, and members of the community in first aid and disaster response.

Natural elements can cause great destruction; it's almost inevitable. However, recovery from natural disasters, like the Haitian earthquake, varies largely depending on the type of destruction, the amount and location of it, and the accessibility of resources to fix the problem. Being part of the "haves" creates a slightly better strategic position to adapt to the changes in the environment wrought by natural forces. But even being part of the elite class, particularly when the infrastructure of the place is lacking, can't always save lives. For the vast majority of those living in Haiti, resources were quite scarce before the quake.

I hadn't been to Port-au-Prince for almost six months, and although it was good to see people carrying on with their day-to-day lives, working, with family, and occasionally smiling, this was far from normal. The tent cities with displaced people, that were supposed to be temporary, were still there and fully occupied. The airport was still undergoing major construction. And seeing the remaining rubble and remnants of buildings more than hinted that there was still a tremendous amount of work that needed to be done.

After a short drive from Toussaint L'Ouverture International Airport, we passed through the metal gates of the Hopital Bernard Mevs. The stone and concrete hospital remained intact and was teeming with patients entering and leaving the buildings. Other buildings had patients seated and lined up waiting to be seen.

After dropping off our bags in our dorm room, which consisted of a series of bunk beds, I scarfed down a Styrofoam container filled with remarkably seasoned rice and beans while meeting with the other delegates. Unlike most of my usual meetings, this one took place outside in the hospital's concrete courtyard. We sat in a circle, much like what would be expected at a summer camp but without the campfire, and discussed Haiti, its past and current state, and the vision of what we could collectively achieve to further develop emergency and trauma care. I thought it was kind of cool having a goal-setting staff meeting sitting outside in front of the hospital, rather than in a stuffy classroom. I also wondered if the reason we were outside was because people still feared spending too much time in buildings, even if they were deemed earthquake-proof.

The next morning the outside circle meetings continued, but the afternoon was dedicated to spending time with the local Haitian physicians and surgeons in the clinical areas of the hospital and emergency department. With the exception of windows allowing light to enter and oval-shaped openings in the outside walls that helped circulate air to cool down the rooms, the emergency department wasn't much different from the ones I was used to back in the US. It still smelled medicinal from the harsh chemicals used to scrub the floors and clean the beds to keep them infection-free. It still had the feel of any emergency department, with people having that same nervous look, not wanting to be there and hoping to get out as quickly as possible. Being sick, or hurt enough to have to go to the emergency department, in any place where people don't have a lot of money means there is a perceived risk of death. I didn't have to be fluent in Haitian Creole to know the specific fears the patients and their families had because the universal stress lines between their eyes and foreheads were clearly evident.

The emergency department at the Hopital Bernard Mevs was a lot quieter than the ones I worked at in Brooklyn, mainly because there weren't patients, techs, and docs yelling across the room. Maybe people in Brooklyn were just loud and I'd been so used to people being loud that moments of quiet and peace seemed out of the ordinary. Trying to make their way through the high volume of patients, the medical staff worked swiftly, seeing patients with a gamut of illnesses and injuries. I didn't see any shortage of medical supplies, but Haiti was still considered a disaster zone, and the hospitals and local businesses had not completely recovered to pre-earthquake standards. Taking this into consideration, everyone knew not to squander supplies needed for patient care in case another catastrophe occurred.

Just like back home, there were kids coming in to be treated for various burns, injuries, and the usual pediatric illnesses like common colds and random rashes that could result from ringworm to bug bites or an allergic reaction. There were adults with asthma attacks and chest pain, and people injured from falling off their motorcycles and scooters.

Things were relatively calm until they weren't. Just like back home, two Black men, both in their twenties, both from a poor Black neighborhood, were brought into the trauma bay after being shot multiple times. Luckily, the bullets had only hit them in the arms and legs, so they were likely to survive. They would now only have to live with the memory of what happened to them that afternoon, almost certainly bearing those psychic scars long after the physical injuries healed.

How the two young men would fare once they were discharged from the hospital would depend to some extent on whether their lived environments would be more forgiving. Given their history and the most recent events, the city and the country hadn't been forgiving and they were likely to remain that way for some time to come. These young men would have a tough time staying safe. The violence was all too familiar, even though this was Haiti.

The whole scenario, in fact, was too familiar. I hadn't wanted to get accustomed to violence, but I already was. I expected it. Just like I expected weather to change during different seasons, I expected violence to happen with warm weather in poor cities with poor Black people, and it bothered me. I didn't welcome it or even want it to come, but here it was again, identical and like clockwork.

I'd cared for more than enough shooting victims and had grown tired of it. The medical staff was still unaware of the circumstances and specific details around the shooting, but as with most patients I'd treated with violent injuries, the speculation over the causes varied from gang violence, self-defense, retaliation, or maybe just plain old robbery. Given the burning tires outside the hospital compound, the violence could have been associated with the upcoming elections, with various parties vying for power and resorting to physical assault.

The immediate cause of the shooting was important for solving a crime, but there were a host of other issues taking place in the country that led to a series of perfect storms, making this shooting just one of many. These weren't accidental injuries brought on solely by a natural disaster but instead were a culmination of factors, including all the attendant ills of poverty, which were greatly exacerbated by the destruction and hardship caused by the quake, the power imbalance, and the great inequity in the social fabric that had prevailed for so long.

If I were a police detective, then evaluating the immediate sequence of events that led to the shooting of the two young men in Port-au-Prince and identifying the one who pulled the trigger might help prevent another shooting by the assailant. But the act of violence was much more problematic than the simple naming of the assailant.

There were things to be assumed: Whoever the shooter was, they deemed their own life more important than the lives they attacked. Whether the shooter shot in defense or preemptively, they were concerned about protecting something they personally thought was important: property, power, or preserving their own survival. If the shooter was a hired gun and had received money to carry out an assassination, the job led to the preservation of their livelihood through financial benefits. If the two men shot were candidates in a local election, or members of a particular political party and they were attacked by the camp of another candidate, the camp of the attacker was either intent on changing a political landscape or preserving a landscape to fit the best interest of that party.

The injuries of the patients, their trauma, was what I was most familiar with. It was most understandable and most visible. I could see the injuries and the pain on the faces of the victims. But it's the invisible damage, the trauma that you don't see, the trauma that haunts you and is re-lived, that keeps you up at night. It's the trauma that creates tension in your relationships because of unresolved issues. It's the vicarious trauma that you pass on to your family and that moves to others in the community. It's the trauma that people have because they have been displaced—forcibly or economically—and live in a place far from their birth home. It's the trauma that comes from living in a place where you don't control the economic development of your community and where you don't feel safe.

I didn't always remember my patients after treating them, but I remembered their eyes and the fear they held onto, not knowing if they would come out alive. That look in the eyes of the two young men on the gurneys in Port-au-Prince was the same.

The injuries of the patients were a mere symptom of what they were already experiencing. The environment in which they were born, and continued to live in, was one of suffering. One could argue that the conditions were solely the result of corrupt government officials who pocketed wealth for themselves and their families and concealed it in foreign bank accounts or offshore investments. But the history of the land, from what had been taken away from its indigenous occupants and their African replacements forced to work the land for their oppressors' benefit, was a major component of the causality of trauma in Haiti.

Understanding Haiti, or better yet the human experience, is to recognize the intersections of the physical with the invisible in the environment. Like many cities and countries around the world, they are often divided into those who have and those who don't. To have, in Haiti, or in other underdeveloped countries, is to be in a position of access: access to goods, education, medical care, and opportunity. To have, means not having to beg for things to care for your family. It means that you can afford medication if you are sick. It means not having to choose between eating, education, and health. It means there is the possibility for mobility and movement beyond the things that bind you to the land or space that you occupy. For those who don't have enough, or much of anything, the struggle is to survive—and even survival isn't a guarantee. The environment doesn't provide; it is merely a space that you occupy.

Both young men had remained stable and had been admitted to the hospital for the further management of their wounds, and the emergency department became calm again. Their futures were full of uncertainty nonetheless.

Eventually the smoke cleared and the protestors outside left. The barricade of burning tires was removed and the driver gave us the thumbs-up that it was OK to leave the compound. We would be able to get to the airport and catch our scheduled flight back, and I would make it in time for work back in Brooklyn, only to face nearly identical cases to those we had just treated in Port-au-Prince.

Over the years, my thinking about violence as a public health issue, and the need for violence prevention programs, has also been shaped by working in underdeveloped countries. I've spent time working in Haiti and Kenya, as well as in Peru, Guyana, and Brazil. The common thread for all of these places, including some of the US, is the blatant evidence of the health disparities, violence, trauma, systemic racism, and colorism fostered by the economic injustice of colonialism.

I treated many diseases of poverty—kwashiorkor, malnutrition, and more. And in Haiti, of course, there was also the aftermath of natural disaster to complicate and inflame the issues. Both experiences were crucibles for me as a young physician. And like my experience in Chicago, they were essential to my understanding of the larger systemic ways that trauma and violence affect a community. I never could have arrived at the understandings I did without my time in each country.

In many ways, the countries I'd worked in couldn't be more different from each other, or from the US. But all have suffered from long histories of colonization—Guyana and Kenya by the British Empire, Brazil by the Portuguese, and Haiti by France. The countries have been robbed of many of their resources and are much more challenged and far more impoverished than they should be given their natural resources. What I began to see in these places is how trauma plays out and how the entire system has to be changed. Improving public health outcomes, in relation to violence or in relation to anything else, means looking at ways to reform the system.

This was where I discovered a responsibility to understand the deep root causes of the issue of violence (of any societal issue, in fact). If I was truly going to contribute to fixing social inequities— whether it be in Kenya, Chicago, Brooklyn, or anywhere else—I needed more than just a professional grasp of disease pathology. I needed to continue to develop a plan that directly addressed those causes, and not just the symptoms. Lack of funding was a roadblock, but the seed was planted and my conviction continued to grow.

CHAPTER 11

DO SOMETHING

WE HAD A GREAT NAME, which was exciting, but I'd have been lying if I had said I was optimistic. I was perpetually burned out, anxious, frustrated and stressed, sometimes all at once. I was still a practicing emergency physician, seeing tons of patients every shift, many of them victims of the violence that I was hoping to curb. There was some comfort in moving forward with an idea, but the problem of failing spectacularly or even not achieving the results we hoped for was unsettling.

Looking back, I think it was because I didn't understand what progress truly meant. People often mistake progress for completion. But after a while, I learned that each small step, when completed and done well, would get us closer to our goal. No matter how stressed I was on the road to success I was on at the time, I came to believe in the end that it was worth it.

Research grants and other types of funding rejections are a lot like college applications or book manuscript submissions: a "no" isn't the end of the world. The world is full of other people ready and willing to help you make your dreams a reality. You must be patient and send out dozens of applications—sometimes hundreds— before you find that person or organization who understands the value you offer. Each grant application had similar questions on what KAVI intended to do, but some wanted to hear about programming for teens, while others wanted information specifically about Black men, Black women, at-risk adults, after-school programs, and so on. Several wanted to know what we were already doing as a program. That was the most irritating because we didn't have a program—that's why we were applying for money!

Rejections were plentiful, but with each application we submitted, our answers seemed better than the previous round. Still feeling impatient, I gradually understood that there were different elements of the program that we hadn't thought through yet, but which were required to properly execute on KAVI's mission. We needed to go through and refine every aspect: identifying, in great detail, the problem that the organization was going to fix, creating the framework for the approach, building the team, putting together the infrastructure to house and maintain the program, locating space, and then, finally, securing resources.

The recurring question in the applications I kept seeing related to what KAVI was already doing. Frankly, the organization only existed on paper. The talks and lectures I was giving to community groups and in academic circles didn't directly relate to my fledgling nonprofit. To make the connection more apparent, a decision was made to do all future advocacy work under the name KAVI. If people didn't know the organization existed, then how could they help support the movement?

The advocacy work we were doing consisted of speaking in front of community groups, elected officials, local news programs, medical conferences, and schools, and that continued for another year and half under the KAVI name. Dr. Austin and I would lead talks to community groups around the city, and the medical students on our team helped do presentations with the Brooklyn district attorney's office. I spoke at national conferences for emergency medicine, forums on violence prevention, at nursing conferences, to community groups, on local news programs, at medical conferences and schools, or to whomever would invite us. The talks were a great way to meet new people who could be helpful allies and garner more support for the movement we were creating. The KAVI name was starting to get out there and I was developing an area of expertise in violence intervention, but we still had no true product other than spreading our new gospel of how to treat victims of violent trauma.

The great thing about growing up in New York City was that, although it's big in size and population, the people are still connected. I had friends in all the boroughs who were involved in everything from the arts, medicine, education, business, and even crime. It wouldn't take much effort to reach out for their help and assistance. A childhood friend, Hank Willis Thomas, had become a prominent and prizewinning visual artist. I always admired his work and since I was making more speeches and had the need for visuals in the presentations, I asked if it was OK to use a picture of one of his pieces that would force people to think differently about violence. Hank graciously agreed so we included the image *Priceless* at my first presentation on violence. In 2000, Hank's cousin, close friend, and roommate, Songha Willis, was killed in a brutal robbery. In a 2019 interview in the *New York Times*, Hank said, "I remember Songha and I joking about being 21 and black and, like, we made it."[1] Just barely—Songha was twenty-eight when he was killed. Hank took a photograph from the funeral service and manipulated it in a way that made a haunting comment on the value of a life and the horror of how many lives are lost to violence every day. The photograph reminds us that every life is truly priceless and that violence cuts too many lives short.

A few years later, after first using Hank's photo, I reached out again. By this time, it was early 2010. I wanted to see about getting Hank's help with developing a photo-based workshop for KAVI. Due to prior commitments, he suggested another photographer and filmmaker, Bayeté Ross Smith, to help work with KAVI. Bayeté and I had also met before as kids and reconnected as adults. Hank and Bayeté, along with fellow artists Chris Johnson and Kamal Smith, had recently created a multimedia video installation masterpiece called *Question Bridge* in 2010. Here's the description from their website:

The Question Bridge: Black Males project is a platform for Black men of all ages and backgrounds to ask and respond to questions about life in America. We created it to stimulate connections and understanding among Black men, but we also wanted to show the diversity of thought, character and identity in the Black male population so rarely seen in American media. In essence, we want to represent and redefine Black male identity in America.[2]

The stated intention of the project didn't align precisely with our hopes for KAVI—it wasn't solely focused on violence prevention—but the storytelling aspect and the encouragement it offered for young Black men to think deeply about their actions and their place in the world was exciting to me and could be used as a valuable tool to incorporate within KAVI. Since most of the victims of violence who came (and still come) into the emergency department were young Black men, leading them to think about their motivations and values might ultimately lead to a shift in self-perception, and that can make a real difference. Bayeté felt that the mission of our still-nascent KAVI was an extension of the work with their project. I felt the same. I've always been a fan of stories. My mother is a master storyteller and used it to teach me and her students. My father is a photographer so I've always been around a lot of images, and I never looked at them and just thought "nice picture." I always wanted to know, "Who's that? What happened?" I wanted to know the whole story.

At a coffee shop near New York University in the spring of 2010, Bayeté and I went back and forth, brainstorming and writing questions that would be pertinent to the mission. The first step in understanding violence and trauma was looking at our own identity. In theory, talking to kids and patients about violence made sense, but if a patient had been gangbangin' their entire teenage or adult life and we had the conversation about not retaliating, would that cause any meaningful change? What were the skill sets they needed to improve their overall quality of life? Or to make a living and remain gainfully employed? How would we even start the conversation about mental health and wellness and trauma? Why would they listen? We kept sketching out ideas and met weekly in person or via phone conference call to be ready with at least a curriculum for KAVI participants. Ultimately, our conversations helped enrich the curriculum that was developed for Question Bridge as well as our approach at KAVI.

It was the early spring of 2011 and the money hadn't come yet, but additional grant proposal rejections did come. There was still an immediate need to start KAVI's work beyond advocacy, but we lacked funding, so we used the opportunity to figure out who would be the ideal candidates for our new team. I reached out to my good friend Jumaane Williams. Jumaane and I went to school together and had known each other since the fifth grade. At the time I contacted him about KAVI he was a relatively new city council member, but since then he's gone on to become one of New York's most promising young politicians, serving as New York City public advocate and running for governor in 2022. After a conversation about our ideas on KAVI as an advocacy group, that spring Jumaane stepped up to the plate and awarded KAVI a five-thousand-dollar grant. There was one problem, though: having government money promised to you and getting access to that money are two very different things.

There was a newly implemented system for dispersing funding that came from the city council. Any city council funding that was to impact health care was now being dispensed by the New York City Department of Health (DOH). With any grant, there is usually a small amount of paperwork to be filled out. Already working for the city at one of its hospitals, I automatically assumed there would be more paperwork if the grant came from the city. I was correct—there was extensive paperwork. I filled out form after form, notarized documents, sent extensive emails, and also had phone calls with representatives from the DOH, but there always seemed to be another layer of red tape. Saba Debesu, a political strategist and one of KAVI's early volunteers, was very skilled at navigating governmental agencies and helped us get through to access our grant, but even she wasn't able get past the excessive red tape. It was hard to walk away from that money, because we really needed it, but the effort required to tap into it made it impossible. So walk away we did.

I didn't even think to go back to Jumaane for help because I assumed he had more important things to take care of. (Mind you, years later he scolded me for not notifying him about the problem.) But at that moment, I felt like the amount of time we spent chasing the grant, five thousand dollars could have been made in a much shorter time frame by doing a series of overtime shifts in the emergency department. Feeling a bit beaten by the whole ordeal, I poured my focus back into working on the curriculum and building the team.

It had been a few months since trying to get that grant when I got a phone call from a woman named Fatima Ashraf. Fatima was a public health expert and a friend of a friend and worked with New York mayor Michael Bloomberg's office on violence intervention. She said, "Let me give you the heads up. There's gonna be a meeting at your hospital about violence intervention and funding. The mayor is going to propose putting violence intervention programs into the hospitals." I said, "Great!" I was excited for the chance; however, there was a "but" coming soon after her statement. "But the programs are going to be CeaseFire," she said. I knew of Cease-Fire. It was based in Chicago and did intervention work using former gang members for community violence mediations. The model was like the work being done out of Oakland and in Boston by other intervention organizations. I respected their work then and still do. But I was furious.

CeaseFire was started in 1999 by an epidemiologist and physician named Gary Slutkin. Dr. Slutkin had spent ten years in Africa, primarily in Uganda, fighting the AIDS crisis. Before that, he worked in San Francisco to fight the resurgent tuberculosis (TB) epidemic. But when he came back to the States, he couldn't get away from another contagion: violence. It seemed clear to him that violence was much like the diseases he had been fighting for so long in the rest of the world. In a 2008 *New York Times Magazine* profile, he told journalist Alex Kotlowitz, "For violence, we're trying to interrupt the next event, the next transmission, the next violent activity. . . . And the violent activity predicts the next violent activity like H.I.V. predicts the next H.I.V. and TB predicts the next TB."[3]

Slutkin's solution was to start CeaseFire (now known as Cure Violence and one of KAVI's current partners) in 1999. Like KAVI, it started small. And like KAVI, CeaseFire used the gold standard for reversing epidemics: interrupt transmission, reduce risk, and change community norms. Transmission, in this case, meant using "violence interrupters," people who knew the streets and often had been involved in violent activities themselves, to talk to people right at the moment they were angriest and most ready to seek revenge and try to talk them out of the retaliation that the "code of the street" demands. People like Willis. To help change someone's behavior in a highly emotional and traumatic time is most arduous, but with persistence these interrupters can become trusted confidants, persuading the injured party that the cost of getting back at someone is just too high, that revenge hurts both parties and leaves only more damage behind. The interrupters also reduce risk. In the same *New York Times Magazine* story, Alex Kotlowitz tells of occasions where violence interruption fails or doesn't achieve all that would be ideal. It doesn't necessarily fend off a crime—but it can fend off a murder. That's part of the reduction of risk and very much what we're working toward at KAVI through our programs in schools (more about that shortly) as well as our hospital interventions. The final step, changing community norms, is the hardest one. Breaking down the code of the street is tough, especially when you're working with people who have been traumatized, in many instances repeatedly, as they are often operating on a hair trigger. Even if they are trained to react differently, sometimes it's hard for folks to push back against not only years of conditioning but years of negative events, as I was to see with Willis.

CeaseFire was on point in its mission. But the leadership was based in Chicago. Chicago and New York City were two different places. To be clear: I will always support any person or organization actively working toward positively transforming the quality of life for Black and Brown people and toward ending violence in our communities. CeaseFire was absolutely doing that in Chicago. My anger came about because I'd been working on my program for years and began wondering if all that time, effort, and knowledge about our specific Brooklyn community was about to be dismissed with the wag of one politician's finger. Blindly supporting this program from another city without exploring efforts already underway closer to home meant the mayor's office was looking for a Band-Aid. They didn't have any idea what was going on already inside their own boundaries.

As with changing any behavior or health issue, particularly interrupting and healing violence, it is of utmost importance to involve the people most impacted by the problem as part of the solution. Fresh ideas from outside of the community can complement what is already being done and developed. But not being aware of what exists, or being developed, can create conflicts and needlessly waste resources, ultimately impacting patient care. When people from the outside have moved on to the next project, those people within an area most impacted by the issue, in this case violence, will be left to fend for themselves. This was something I came to understand working abroad and it applied in Brooklyn. The treatment of violence needed comprehensive community leadership that understood the health system, the patients, and the community. I knew the hospital and how it worked. We were already building alliances with community groups and religious leaders in the area. I knew Brooklyn. We just needed some fiscal support.

My anger over KAVI being ignored made me want to skip the meeting altogether, but I got smart and dragged myself there anyway. There were a number of powerful suits from Kings County Hospital, some from the other parts of NYC Health + Hospitals (the country's largest conglomerate of public hospitals, of which Kings County Hospital is a part), and a bunch of folks from the mayor's office, among them Deputy Mayor Linda Gibbs, who was in charge of health.

With the exception of one person from the mayor's office, a delegate from Harlem Hospital, another delegate from Queens

Hospital, executive director Tony Martin of Kings County Hospital, Dr. Austin, and me, everyone else in the room of close to forty people was white. However, in 2011 in New York City 61.8 percent of murder victims were Black, 26.3 percent were Latino, and only 8.4 percent were white.[4] The key players in that room, representing millions of dollars in logistical and legislative power, were talking about issues of systemic violence in the Black and Brown community, with only a handful of the voices in the room actually from that community. The team from CeaseFire at the meeting was also predominantly white. The folks on stage, as well as those participating in the video conference call from Chicago, were mostly white.

I had a lot of questions. Did the meeting organizers recognize or particularly care if their team was balanced? Did the word *representation* come up in their planning meeting, or was it an afterthought? CeaseFire presented the scope of their program. They had a testimonial from their newly launched hospital program at Christ Hospital in Chicago. It was a skillful presentation—but I was still salty about KAVI being ignored. As the meeting appeared to be wrapping up, Kings County's executive director Tony Martin spoke up and gave us our due. Within a few seconds of the end of CeaseFire's presentation, he interjected, "Well, we've had some people in our own hospital that have been working on stuff for a while without support, and I think you might want to hear from them."

I'd been making speeches and giving presentations since high school, and I'd been out in these streets banging the drum for KAVI for a few years. But I didn't expect to get called on in a meeting like this. I would often get a twisting sensation in my stomach prior to a presentation. By forcing myself to present even more over the years, as a student, a doctor, and now as a leader, I was learning to quell fear when I was called to talk. All of those conference presentations—prepared and impromptu talks at gatherings and random meetings, discussing my platform—had been prep work for this moment.

As Mr. Martin introduced me, I could see some sheepish looks coming from the team from the mayor's office and CeaseFire staff.

Not gonna lie—it made me laugh a little inside to see their discomfort. But that wasn't the important thing. I had to make sure that everyone could completely feel what was at stake and that the about-to-be-born KAVI was the organization for the job. So I did the most logical thing I could think of to stay cool and channel that sense of urgency. I started humming Eminem's song "Lose Yourself," in my head, the lyrics talked about having only one shot and not blowing this one opportunity, which helped me remain calm and focused.

I told my story from Brooklyn to Chicago and back, the insights learned from both cities, the connections and the differences between CeaseFire's and KAVI's respective missions. I spoke as someone from the community, actively working in it, about the need to have a successful mission, not solely to decrease community violence but to promote health and community well-being as well. I believed in KAVI, and I knew it would be effective once it launched, but the presence of CeaseFire meant we had to form some sort of synergistic relationship with a competing philosophy. Dr. Austin and Mr. Martin both smiled at me. The years of investing in their mentee had paid off. (Later in the meeting it was disclosed that the potential CeaseFire groups were Brooklyn-based organizations, Man Up! Inc. and SOS, which used the CeaseFire model but were independent groups based in Black neighborhoods and with Black leadership. This eased my anxiety substantially about having people from another city working in Brooklyn. Over the years, working closely together with Man Up! Inc., SOS, and more recently another organization using the CeaseFire model called G-MACC [Gangstas Making Astronomical Community Changes], we have built a special and comprehensive violence intervention blueprint that has benefited the Brooklyn community as a whole.)

For a few minutes all I heard was a deafening silence (it was probably only a few seconds). After a few whispers, one voice spoke up. It was Deputy Mayor Gibbs. "We apologize," she said. "We had no idea that you were doing anything like this here, but we will see how we can help support your efforts."

CHAPTER 12

THE MANY FACES OF VIOLENCE

THE RED NOTIFICATION PHONE RANG in the critical care and trauma (CCT) emergency department on a chilly spring morning with its old-school analog ring. On the other end of the phone, the EMS dispatcher was letting us know that there was a trauma notification coming in with an estimated time of arrival of five minutes. The patient was a twenty-something-year-old woman who had been assaulted and had a head injury with loss of consciousness.

It was pretty early in the day for a violent trauma, but it was the weekend and whatever was coming in could have lingered from the night before. Though there were certain patterns of behavior and types of emergencies that were influenced by time—such as the increased stretchers filled with inebriated people on holidays like Labor Day weekend or right after the ball dropped on New Year's and more elderly people coming into the ED on Sundays after church (after getting dizzy and lightheaded and passing out, as Sunday was their only day to leave the house and a natural stress test)—anything was possible pretty much anytime. Borrowing from science fiction author Frank Herbert, "Deep in the human unconscious is a pervasive need for a logical universe that makes sense. But the real universe is always one step beyond logic."[1] The ED was anything but logical.

Whenever possible, EMS called the ED if they were bringing in a patient with serious injuries, meaning there was a high probability of death or the potential for a critical problem like an intracranial hemorrhage (aka brain bleed) or long-term harm, like losing a limb. This way, the team was able to prepare the equipment needed for the incoming patient and notify the appropriate services (respiratory therapy, trauma surgery, orthopedic surgery, or anesthesia). This was done in what was described as the "golden hour of trauma," when diagnosis, intervention, and treatment initiated within the first hour of severe injury would increase the chances of the patient surviving and doing well.

Within five minutes of receiving the notification, EMS brought in a Black woman wearing a cervical spine collar and with obvious signs of head injury consisting of multiple bruises and scrapes to the face, and congealed blood covering her wig. We noted quickly that she was transgender. She was in serious condition but stable, as her vital signs were within normal limits and she was breathing OK and speaking coherently.

"I got jumped, by some guys," she told us. She didn't offer any information as to the circumstances of how or why she got jumped, but I guessed that it was either a random robbery or a hate crime. With any trauma, the initial goal was to rule out any critical injuries and provide the most effective and timely treatment. Once the patient was stable, and while they were being worked up, it was appropriate to investigate causes of the trauma and make sure there was a safety plan to mitigate harm from happening in the future. This could be especially important in the case of a hate crime.

Our medical team ordered the appropriate bloodwork, CT scans, and X-rays and later repaired the scalp lacerations. I'd seen too many traumas to count, but despite their familiarity I was always shocked at the brutality one person could inflict on another and disappointed in humanity's prehistoric continuity of violence. All of the CT scans were negative, and fortunately the bruises and scalp laceration scars would heal and she would fully recover from the injuries. But surviving the trauma would be a different matter, and I always worried if the injured person, particularly one so vulnerable, would come back with more injuries, perhaps more severe ones, down the road.

While walking over to the patient's room, one of the nurses pulled me aside and said that the area where the patient had been assaulted had a high number of prostitutes. I hadn't even considered that the patient might be a sex worker injured by a client or a pimp; I didn't want to assume the woman was a sex worker, but I couldn't remove the possibility from the equation, though the fact that she'd been assaulted by a group of men in an area with extensive prostitution made it seem likely. Sex workers have a 45 percent to 75 percent chance of experiencing violence at work.[2]

Exploring other causes of her trauma, I considered the event might be a hate crime targeting the transgender Black woman, as she said that she didn't know the people who kicked and punched her. It wasn't the first time I'd taken care of a transgender woman who had been attacked and beaten. I didn't see these attacks often at our hospital but knew that the trans community experiences high levels of gender-based violence compared to the general population, and up to 89 percent have reported experiencing physical violence.[3] Transgender adults have a higher risk of employment discrimination compared to their cisgender counterparts. They also have higher odds of disability, poor mental health, subjective memory problems, poor physical health, and income below the US poverty level compared to cisgender adults.[4] Transgender persons report double the rates of sexual violence compared to cisgender LGBQ people in a study on lifetime prevalence of sexual assault.[5] What's more, Black and Latina transgender women are at higher risk for hate crimes compared to white transgender women.[6]

I didn't have any transgender friends until relatively recently, when I met one of my new Brazilian jiu-jitsu (BJJ) training partners. She was a great training partner, but we had never spoken about her plight and trauma as a trans woman. I did wonder how she came to make the decision to fully live as a woman, or if she had a gender-affirmation surgery that allowed her to transition into her self-identified gender. In BJJ class my focus was to learn how to execute takedowns, chokes, and submissions and to avoid being submitted while training or sparring. Thinking about things other than what I was doing while training was a sure way to get injured. But I don't think I was comfortable even asking her questions. However, I did read some of her social media posts that described the continued hurt and lingering effects of being a trans person, the discrimination she experienced, and the impact of being a target.

It didn't occur to me until later that one of the people who assaulted my transgender patient might be in the waiting room. I've learned, though, that it wasn't uncommon for the perpetrator to accompany the survivor to the ED. As sick as it sounds, they may have come to the ED with the victim to get them treated, as a way of protecting their asset, much in the same way a person would treat a service animal or a human slave.

Within a few moments, I walked into the room to give the patient the news of her CT scans and X-rays and to gather information about her safety and inquire more about the nature of her assault, but she was gone and had apparently left without being signed out by anyone on the medical staff. She was effectively a "walkout during evaluation," having gone with a person from the waiting room. All that was left was the pulled IV and bloodied hospital sheets, clumped on the stretcher.

Years before, during one of my many orientations at the start of medical school and then again at the start of clinical rotations, we learned about hospital and clinic protocols, interviewing and caring for patients, mandated reporting to police and social service agencies, and ensuring that the patients we cared for were safe after discharge. It was drilled into my head to screen for domestic violence, which had recently been changed to be called intimate partner violence (IPV) because the perpetrator didn't always have to be someone that the victim lived with. IPV can be defined as abuse or aggression (physical or psychological), physical violence, stalking, or sexual violence that occurs among intimate partners, which can include current or past spouses, dating partners, or sexual partners.[7] The change in the name was an important shift in attitudes toward violence to be more inclusive. In medical school, we were taught not to miss the opportunity to engage and possibly to intervene and hopefully to assist with patient safety.

My first emergency medicine research in medical school focused on screening for IPV in the ED. Screening for IPV can be done when taking the patient's social history, which includes asking about any type of behavior that could influence and impact health and well-being, such as where the patient lives and their personal habits (sexual activity, smoking, drinking, and the use of any other mood-altering substance), as well as the behaviors of others in the household. Screening for IPV also includes questions about work or school and the home environment. Who lives at home with a patient is important because their personal habits, along with their support (or lack thereof), impact a patient's ability to be compliant with treatment, including staying on recommended diets, exercise routines, and even bathing. If a patient has no assistance in the home, the likelihood they will come to the hospital or clinic for scheduled follow-up appointments, take their prescribed medications, adhere to recommended diets, and relinquish toxic and harmful habits is much lower, as is their ability to heal from an illness or injury or recover from surgery. Asking these social questions with the hopes of identifying additional risk factors can lead to much better outcomes and possibly save a life.

Asking any person questions about potential, or existing abuse, and identifying that a form of abuse has taken place can be the first step in saving their life, and in recent decades asking about violence has gone from being taboo to being mandated in medical settings. If a patient we are caring for has a bruise or strange mark on them that looks as if it was inflicted by an object or a hand or fist, we, as future healthcare practitioners, should ask about it. Signs of violence can be subtle. There can be physical signs of injury hidden under the clothes. That is one of the reasons we are told to have our patients get undressed and into a gown as part of a comprehensive physical exam, regardless of the chief complaint that brought them to the hospital or clinic. Sometimes there are no physical injuries but the abuse is verbal and easily as frightening and damaging. According to the CDC's National Intimate Partner and Sexual Violence Survey, "Almost 1 in 2 women and more than 2 in 5 men reported experiencing contact sexual violence, physical violence, and/or stalking victimization by an intimate partner at some point in their lifetime."[8]

Since there is no sure way to identify a victim or survivor of violence, it is important to screen patients coming into the emergency department regardless of their chief complaint. This is an additional way to get important information from the patient with the ultimate goal of ensuring the patient is safe and free from harm. When EDs first started screening for IPV, only women were screened. It was purely biased at the time, but now many US emergency departments screen for partner violence regardless of gender, sexual orientation, or expression.

Today, some emergency medicine staffs are better educated about and receive more practice at asking the patient questions about violence that go beyond understanding only the present physical injury, including questions like: "Do you feel safe at home?" "Has anyone that you know or don't know tried to hurt you or harm you?" "Have they tried to force you to do something you didn't want to do?" "Were there any children harmed?" "Have you contacted the police?" "Do you have a safe place to go to?" These are the same questions that can be asked of anyone coming in to an ED with any kind of intentional injury or assault.

IPV was something initially viewed as occurring to women, with men being the perpetrators. However, other groups of people, like same-sex partners, weren't being considered. Until very recently, when two women or two men were injured in an altercation, they were considered two people fighting, rather than being in a possible domestic or partner dispute. The concept of partner violence occurring within transgender relationships, or between cis and trans people, wasn't even discussed. With an enhanced understanding of the impact of trauma, both physical and psychological, proper screening and early recognition of the signs and presentation of partner violence should be an important part of our training of doctors, nurses, and social workers, as well as violence intervention specialists.[9]

I'd known that the faces of violence survivors and victims were part of a spectrum, but not considering the multifaceted plight of my transgender patient early on made me miss an opportunity to assist an injured patient from a highly vulnerable community, one that was regularly subjected to violence. I could only hope that she didn't come back in worse condition or dead.

Today, at KAVI, and in many other violence prevention and treatment organizations, we train our staff to be attentive to the very real possibility of partner violence within the LGBTQIA+ community and to look for the signs of hate crimes against people from that community as well as other marginalized and under-supported communities.

Although the department of social work at Kings County provides the bulk of support for partner violence survivors, there is a fine line between partner violence, sexual violence, and interpersonal violence. It is important that KAVI team members have an understanding and working knowledge of major forms of violence and conflict. Because KAVI provides support to survivors of interpersonal violence at Kings County Hospital, we are able to take advantage of the required training for any employee at our hospital. Some of this includes training on implicit bias, equality versus equity, suicide prevention, partner violence, and working with members of the LGBTQIA+ community, to name a few. The trainings are a combination of digital and online modules as well as in-person lectures and workshops. Some are provided by KAVI's own staff and consultants; some are provided by social workers, behavioral health specialists, and emergency physicians.

I'm part of Kings County Hospital's Department of Emergency Medicine and KAVI has a close relationship with the department, which has provided the nonprofit with additional support and a plethora of partners. One such partner is the Clinical Forensic Medicine Fellowship. Run by Drs. Brigette Alexandra, Elias Yousef, and Keesandra Agenor, the fellowship was created to help emergency personnel develop the "ability to be trauma-informed, patient-centric, and culturally sensitive when interacting with patients."[10] As a partner with the Clinical Forensic Medicine Fellowship (whose members also oversee and coordinate the hospital's Sexual Abuse Response Team program for survivors of sexual violence), KAVI receives in-person training to better recognize patterns of sexual violence, partner violence, and other forms of abuse, thus enhancing the clinical abilities and spectrum of our team with the end goal of providing more in-depth patient care. This kind of training is invaluable and deserves to be widely funded nationwide.

CHAPTER 13

THE KAVI WAY

AFTER THAT MEETING in the late spring of 2011, not wanting to wait any longer for funding, I decided to launch KAVI using a volunteer-based model. It wouldn't be a perfect or a permanent model, but I needed to start somewhere. I'd helped build sustainable medical training programs in Haiti, building relationships within communities in the northern part of the country and with little to no resources, so why couldn't I do something back in Brooklyn?

Since 2011, KAVI has grown substantially with the help of volunteers, paid staff, donations from community members and others, and funding from both the government and private foundations.

Our programs at KAVI are multipronged. Though the initial idea for KAVI was to provide services in the ED, I had an idea that focused even more on public health. What if we worked with people who were at risk *before* they became patients? The first program we launched was at the Wingate High School campus at the High School for Public Service (Wingate has multiple high schools located on its campus), which was across the street from Kings County Hospital. KAVI would be working with kids in school and in the classroom, before they could get into serious trouble with greater, life-altering consequences.[1] The majority of the students were referred to us by the school as people who had histories of frequent fighting, bullying, gang involvement, and poor academic records.

Within a month of launching the school program, we started our hospital intervention program, which focused on patients who were victims, survivors, and even perpetrators of intentional violence. Sometimes people who initiated the violent incident come to the hospital injured and are seen as patients. The story about who initiated the event doesn't always come out until much later. The participants we would see were patients being treated in the ED for violent injuries as well as patients admitted to trauma surgery for further treatment and management.

In 2022, our KAVI hospital team worked with 292 clients who were survivors of violence. What these patients experienced went beyond the physical pain of their injuries; the fresh act of violence, the most recent injury, even hospitalization triggered emotions from old injuries, old hurt, old harsh experiences, and their preexisting trauma. This was the moment when they felt most vulnerable, when they most needed support and guidance. The violent wounds we see aren't always from disputes; we see plenty of innocent bystanders come in injured as well. But whatever the cause, the pain and trauma of violent injury is real and, just like any other disease, needs to be addressed when it happens. Ignoring the nonphysical trauma only allows it to fester and grow. Often when patients are admitted, they are abruptly deprived of the way they manage the ongoing, unacknowledged anxiety that many of them experience. A lot of our patients self-medicate with weed and alcohol to block painful emotions and, even if it doesn't rise to the level of clinical addiction, it's a dependence that, when suddenly removed, increases their suffering and agitation.

No two patients are identical and there are layers and layers of trauma that exist, making treating it more challenging and more complex. Medical staff in the hospital address the physical injuries, but the invisible trauma wouldn't be treated if it weren't for the KAVI violence intervention team and our in-hospital community partners who are part of that team (Man Up! Inc., SOS, G-MACC, the Fortune Society). They understand the lives and worlds of our patients, often having grown up in the same neighborhoods or in a similar one nearby. Here are the stories of a couple of our best.

BENNIE AND SHAH

I met Bennie in the pediatric emergency department in 2011 after he brought his son in for treatment from a dog bite. Happily, the bite to the leg was stable and there were unlikely to be complications. It was a quiet day so I had a little time to talk, and Bennie was eager to find out more about me.

"You're really the doctor?" he said smiling. "We don't see too many Black doctors around, so we're glad you're here. Means a lot in this neighborhood especially."

We chatted for a while about growing up in Brooklyn, about gentrification and about what it was like for him to be raising two sons as a single father. Both boys came in with him and their respect for their father was clear. It was (and still is) very rare to see a father come into the ED with his kids so Bennie stood out in that way as well. Though he was a stranger to the unit, Bennie spoke to the nurses, ER techs, and clerks with ease.

As we talked, I noticed that Bennie had a scar across the left side of his face. It wasn't the kind of scar left by an accident or mishap. It was one of the "buck fifty" scars. When I asked him about it, he chuckled and said "that was from another life when I ran the streets."

Though he was older than most of the patients injured, he seemed like he might be the kind of person we needed as KAVI came to life. I took a chance right then and there and asked if he'd be willing to work with KAVI once we got on our feet. Without hesitation, he said he'd be happy to help. Even though KAVI was little more than an idea, we had our first eager volunteer to do hospital interventions.

Part of what made Bennie a good fit for this role was his life history. One of five brothers, he had been out in the streets himself as a younger man. As we got to know each other and I learned more of his story, I found out that he had been shot five times and was in a knife fight that had led to his scar. He'd also had a long period of depression when he used drugs himself. By the time I met him, he had begun to clean up his act and walk the straight and narrow for his boys. He was working as a chef for the New York City Department of Education and teaching kids in various schools about healthy eating. His pattern of reaching out to the community was well established before I met him.

A few months after Bennie and I met, I was working the 3 to 11 p.m. shift in the CCT area of the ED. This would be Bennie's first time shadowing me in the hospital. Shadowing was a way for him to get familiar with being in the ED—meeting staff, understanding the flow, and getting comfortable being around sick and injured people, especially what we call level 1 traumas. Level 1 codes are those patients who require immediate attention, as determined by the type of injury, the location of the injury, the patient's mental status, clinical presentation, and vital signs (blood pressure, respiratory rate, heart rate). A lot of the people KAVI works with do come in as level-1 trauma codes; however, even if a person's injuries aren't severe, that doesn't negate the need for intervention and support after an act of violence. KAVI's participants are victims of intentional violence, shootings, stabbings, beatings—all the bad things that people are capable of. Once Bennie officially began to volunteer with KAVI, his job title was "violence intervention specialist," a term we borrowed from Caught in the Crossfire, a Youth ALIVE! program in Oakland. As an intervention specialist he would meet with the patient and their family in the ED as soon as the patient was somewhat stable, advocate on behalf of the patient, find out what happened to cause the violent event, determine if retaliation might occur, and see if he could prevent retaliation through persuasion and peer counseling. It was a lofty task but much needed.

It was important that an intervention and support would be available immediately after a person experienced a trauma. Early intervention—especially during the golden hour of trauma—can improve the overall survival for the trauma patient. When I began to do specific research and learn about intentional trauma and violence as a public health problem, I came across the work of Dr. Carnell Cooper, a trauma surgeon in Maryland who started a violence intervention program in Baltimore simply called Violence Intervention Program (VIP), which was a model for KAVI. Dr. Cooper described his work in a 2011 interview with the *New York Times*:

In trauma surgery, we refer to the time from injury to getting the patient to the hospital as "the golden hour." We've started to call our prevention work the second golden hour because it's a second opportunity to save lives.

When these young people are in the hospital in pain, with tubes coming out of every orifice, and their mother, father, girlfriend around the bed crying, it may be the first time this person has had a chance to pause and reconsider things. And it's an opportunity for us to ask questions and get things moving forward. In jail, people are just trying to survive, to be tough and get out. In the hospital, they are in a safe environment, one that affords them the opportunity to have a little bit of perspective. We're simply trying to take advantage of that opportunity.[2]

I modeled the vision for KAVI on this idea.

Bennie was shadowing me in the ED, and this was his very first day. Shortly after we arrived at the CCT, a sixteen-year-old boy came in with serious injuries after being beaten by grown men. He had been kicked, punched, and hit with blunt objects until he was a pulp. His eyes were swollen shut. His face was disfigured and his arms, legs, and body were swollen and bruised. The boy, named Shah, didn't have any beef with anyone in particular, but his family did. Before the beating, a member of his extended family had shot and killed someone, creating a feud between the families that never faded away. For months now, retaliatory violence had been going back and forth between the two warring families. Shah was caught in the middle. He loved to skateboard but was small for his age—which made him stand out and made him an easy target.

After his preliminary assessment, we could see that Shah would survive his injuries, but I was afraid that this incident would escalate the war between the families. It wasn't long before his parents arrived to see their son beaten to a minimally recognizable state. His parents were fuming, understandably so, and pacing back and forth as I explained their son's injuries and the next course of action. Part of their reaction included remarks like "We know what we have to do next." This made it clear that the battle was still raging, that Shah's family was pledging war. I continued to speak to them, offering support and any answers I could provide, running the gamut of talking to them about Shah's aftercare and the need for them to be wise and safe, but I could feel their anger rising. At the same time, new clinical emergencies arrived in the ED that needed my immediate attention and I had to excuse myself politely but abruptly. This is a regular thing in emergency medicine life. No sooner have you dealt with one complex problem or patient then you're on to the next one.

But Shah's family still needed help. Even though Bennie was new to the ED, I trusted that his lived experience would guide him and gave him a look. Our mutual understanding began that day. I introduced Bennie to the family as our "violence intervention specialist," and he immediately began to talk with the family members, listening, guiding, and persuading them away from violent retaliation.

Bennie spent close to eight hours with the parents and other family and friends coming in to visit Shah. He was so relaxed and comfortable that he managed to guide the distraught family members to calm down and even got them to smile a little bit in the midst of this awful situation. Bennie was able to spend enough time with them so they could articulate their fears and concerns and ask plenty of questions, however repetitive they may have been (people have a tendency to repeat questions during emergencies because of anxiety). Bennie was a model of patience, listening calmly and turning to the ED team for support when necessary. When it was time to leave, the family thanked Bennie and the rest of our team for being patient with them and even apologized for suggesting that someone in their family would harm another person in retaliation.

That night with Bennie set the precedent for the type of support KAVI was going to offer. And for Bennie, it was the beginning of, as he puts it, his path in life. He worked with us until 2010 when he left to focus on his own wellness and education. He went to college, got certified as a peer counselor, and rejoined us as a full-time staff member in 2022. He's helped hundreds of people and has saved and changed hundreds of lives. When I asked him what was most effective when working with the trauma patients and families he said, "I focus on their mental wellness. You have to get past that ego—that 'naw man, I'm alright, I'm alright'—to find out what's really going on. I'll be talking to somebody and there's a loud noise and they jump up and that's when I'm like, 'See, you're triggered.' Once they admit that, then we can talk."

TAISHA AND DIVINE

Taisha came to us through Man Up! Inc., a partner organization that was founded by her uncle, Brother A. T. Mitchell. KAVI works with several nonprofits to broaden our reach, so Taisha was working at Kings County as an employee of Man Up! Inc. We were so impressed by her care for and skill with patients that we were happy to welcome her aboard when funding for a full-time position became available. Taisha doesn't hide her past: when she was twenty-one, she was incarcerated for six and a half years for assault with a deadly weapon. But surviving through that time and trying to offer a kind of restitution for those she hurt is part of what drives her today. "I did damage to my community," she says now, "and this is my way to give back, even though I wasn't able to reach my victims and those I hurt. I got my GED, I went to college, I did advocacy so that we could get the tools we needed for our classwork. When I was inside, I had to decide to do the time and not let the time do me."

We benefit from her efforts to "do the time" productively every day. One of Taisha's gifts is the subtlety with which she can read a patient's body language and calibrate her approach to where they're at emotionally in the wake of injury. "Once I go into the room, it feels like I just smell the air in the room—not literally but in terms of how this might go. I look closely at their facial expressions and then I can see how to reach past the barriers they might have up." She uses the same approach to help calm distressed family members, managing their heightened emotions, which sometimes come out in the form of anger or abusiveness.

Taisha works as a violence intervention specialist and is also a member of KAVI's hospital intervention team, helping patients navigate potential obstacles once they're discharged and guiding them to the services they need. She also helps them begin to understand the nature of the experience they've just been through. Here's how she puts it:

> Often, they don't look at their experience as trauma until you bring it up to them. In this community this stuff is sometimes passed off as "oh yeah, well, things happen. This is just part of everyday life." So when I talk to them and start breaking it down, they start to get it. They start to understand that this kind of thing they go through really isn't normal, isn't something you can go through without reaction. This shouldn't be a part of everyday life. When you get out of here, for example, you might be reactive to loud noises. But we've equipped you to know what's going on and to have better tools to deal with it.

Taisha and the team are there for the patients for a minimum of one year after their injuries. However, services are provided as long as needed. We have been working with some clients for over three years. We help the participants secure physical therapy needs, employment, even housing as necessary. Our case managers get to know who they're working with and help them find what they need to move forward. We can't get everyone yet, but each life we touch matters.

One such life is Derek "Divine," who appears in the documentary *Trauma and Treatment: How Violence Interrupters Help Heal*, part of a trilogy of documentaries called *The Damage Done* produced by BRIC TV here in Brooklyn.[3] Divine was hanging out with some friends on Christmas Eve, doing nothing in particular, when suddenly he heard a blast and found himself on the ground, shot through the leg. His leg was nearly blown apart, requiring a series of "excruciating, excruciating" surgeries. He made it through, and we were there every step of the way, helping him find housing and getting him into physical rehab right away. "What they did was spectacular," says Derek. "Once they told me I could put weight on my leg, they had me out of there in seventy-two hours." But Derek still feels the mental impact of the trauma and suffers from nightmares—"head on a swivel," as he puts it. Taisha and the team are working to support him through that too. KAVI does that for several hundred patients each year.

MOE

Moe was nineteen when he came to Kings County, months after being shot in the back during a gang altercation in the Bronx where he lived. His injuries were severe, damaging his spinal cord and leaving him paralyzed from the waist down. After his initial wounds were treated at a hospital in the Bronx, his road to recovery and long-term rehabilitation—adjusting to life with his new paralysis—would prove slow. He started in Manhattan with intensive physical and occupational therapy for a few months and then moved to Brooklyn for subacute rehabilitation with less intensive therapy to help him learn how to perform his regular activities of daily living while being confined to a wheelchair. While in subacute rehab, he developed urinary tract and pelvic infections, leading to problems with his kidneys, at which point he came to Kings County Hospital for immediate medical intervention. If his infection went untreated, he would die relatively quickly. Moe was referred to KAVI because of the nature of his initial injuries. His infection eventually subsided, but his paralysis remained.

The first time Bennie and I visited him in his hospital room, he pulled the sheet over his head and turned away. He wasn't ready to speak with us, so we left, gently adding that we would come back. This routine would happen a few times before he finally spoke to the team. Moe was clearly in pain. Not just from his wounds or the infections but from the deep pain that comes from losing physical freedom.

Prior to his transfer to Kings County, Moe had already received treatment for his injuries for more than six months. I understood his anger and his short temper. For weeks on end, strange people donning masks and gowns and smelling of sanitizer came into his room daily to clean him, serve food, and give him medications before leaving his hospital room as quickly as possible. The depersonalization of the interactions was exacerbated by the added need for sterility in the midst of the COVID pandemic, making the hospital even more impersonal than normal. He'd also been hardened growing up in the Bronx and feeling the need to protect himself at all times. Anything new and unfamiliar was suspicious.

I am not a nurse, but I work with them daily. Nursing happens to be one of the toughest and most frequently underappreciated professions; without them our patients would die. Period. Nurses work unbelievably hard and receive a lot of anger directed at them from doctors, surgeons, administrators, families, and patients, mainly because they spend the most time with the patients and are therefore an easy target. Nurses are often tired, stressed, and frequently overworked, making it understandable that sometimes their reserves of compassion run low. Refusing his meds and yelling at nurses gave Moe a bad rep. Along with his nurses, his physical therapists and even social workers labeled him "noncompliant" and had a difficult time placing him in a subacute rehab facility. The language used to describe Moe was a clear indication that the nurses had their own preexisting traumas and were triggered by interactions with him. Moe was traumatized and the nurses were traumatized—not an ideal matchup.

As a patient, Moe exhibited the patterns of grieving delineated by Dr. Elisabeth Kübler-Ross, a Swiss American psychiatrist whose work focused on the study of near-death patients and their mental processes. Her groundbreaking book *On Death and Dying* outlines five stages of grief that occur in someone with a terminal illness.[4] (Moe wasn't dying, but the loss and adjustments that he was experiencing were comparable to those of someone with a terminal illness.) The first stage is *denial*, where the person is unable to accept or believe the trauma or illness that has taken place. They might even describe feeling numb to what has happened to them. The second is *anger*, which can typically manifest as subtly as feeling irritated or extra annoyed by trivial things but which can also show up more intensely as violent outbursts. The third is *bargaining*, often described as the "what if" stage. *What if I avoided hanging out with a certain crowd? Could my problems have been avoided? If I volunteer my time and strive to be a better person, would my injuries heal?* The fourth stage is *depression*, a mood disorder that can be described as having periods of intense sadness, impacting a person's interests, actions, and how they view the world and engage with their day-to-day responsibilities. As humans we have the ability to experience a variety of emotions, but when the emotion takes over and prohibits us from being able to work, go to school, eat, or focus, then that sadness is considered pathologic. The fifth and final stage is *acceptance*, the act of acknowledging that loss has taken place or is inevitable. Acceptance does not mean that the person is OK with the loss but they understand that the loss exists. The stages aren't completely linear or cyclical. They don't have a set time where they should resolve. Some can last seconds, while others may last weeks or even years. Some stages may even occur concurrently.

Through the almost daily check-ins with Bennie and other intervention team members during his months of hospitalization, Moe eventually began to open up. Bennie would bring food from outside the hospital for him and would just sit with him, sometimes trying to get him to laugh, sometimes just sitting in the chair in his room without saying anything. When given permission by the hospital, Bennie took him outside in a wheelchair to get some fresh air and feel the sun.

These gestures made a tangible impact. Having a person just be present, without judgment and whose sole job was to listen and hear him assisted in his healing. Moe went on to make friends during his time in rehab and would take them to meet Bennie. A practicing Muslim, Moe returned to his daily prayers and even extended himself to helping feed two quadriplegic men he befriended in subacute rehab. Through association and resocialization, he was able to reimagine his life as more than the limits placed on his body. By giving him space to process what he was dealing with, he was able to grieve, and he couldn't engage with the complicated task of continuous living until he was able to go through his stages of grieving.

Several months passed before I would have an actual face-to-face conversation and interaction with Moe, who by this time was in a subacute rehab facility near the hospital. We spoke outside in the cool fall air while he smoked some weed (it's legal in New York). He smiled and joked and spoke about his future and wanting to finish high school to go to college to study either business or computer science, but making sure that he did some work to help people who lived in poverty, the way his parents grew up in West Africa. Prior to his being shot when he was in the eleventh grade, he had been on track to graduate on time.

Moe's hospitalization was prolonged by recurrent infections, some of which were due to antibiotic resistance, but also exacerbated by his occasional refusal to take his daily medications. He had been labeled as a problem patient and although his infections eventually healed, he wasn't able to move back home; he was technically homeless. His parents didn't live together. His father's building wasn't wheelchair accessible. He had a challenging relationship with his mother and, because he had verbally abused her before his injuries, wasn't allowed to live with her. With KAVI supporting him, Moe is now working to confront the challenges he has with his mother and other family members and to live on his own. Moe is currently back in high school and actively working toward getting his diploma.

JAVAUN

KAVI has so many great stories about its work against violence, but one of my favorites is this one about a twenty-two-year-old immigrant.

Javaun arrived in our emergency department by ambulance after receiving a life-threatening stab wound to his neck. It turned out he had been stabbed by someone he knew, someone who had been a friend. A drug deal involving marijuana went sour and Javaun's associate, his former friend, and their crew jumped him. He was punched and kicked and fought back; but someone had a knife and stabbed him during the fracas. He didn't even realize that he had been stabbed until he saw blood dripping from his neck onto his body and the ground.

His injuries were stabilized immediately by the emergency team, but, given the location of his injuries, a level-1 trauma code was called to mobilize the trauma team and other surgical subspecialties to assist with his care and management. After a series of diagnostic studies, he was found to have an injury to his carotid artery, which required him to have emergency surgery.

While the emergency medicine and trauma team were caring for Javaun's physical wounds, Taisha had also been alerted. Her pager had gone off at the same time the level-1 trauma code was called and she was at his bedside within minutes. Taisha's role was also essential to saving Javaun's life by providing emotional support, advocating on his behalf, and making sure there was no retaliatory violence. During emergencies, the doctors and surgeons spend time with the patients finding out the history relevant to diagnose and treat. The nurses spend a lot more time administering medications, placing IVs, monitoring the patient, and keeping an extensive record of the patient's evolving condition. There's not a lot of time for the medical team to sit with the patient and listen to and address their immediate and long-term fears, which may be tied to their injury or even preexisting health conditions. Taisha's sole purpose was to talk to Javaun, to find out how he was feeling emotionally and psychologically, and to determine what he needed to be more comfortable. Her role also involved easing Javaun's anxiety at finding himself in a hospital with a life-threatening injury, amid the cacophony of loud bells, beeps from monitors, yelling of the staff issuing orders, and calling in consultants. Taisha's calm presence was essential. Although it was important for her to determine some of the reasons why Javaun was stabbed, to help troubleshoot and ensure there was no retaliatory violence, that conversation would happen later. The immediate issue was to get Javaun to surgery to repair the injured blood vessels, but he was resistant.

He was obviously scared; he could have died from the injuries to his neck and his fear and skepticism about the trauma team and their motives was high. He was even skeptical about the KAVI team and their motive. The ice was broken after Taisha asked him if he needed us to call his family so that they knew he was OK. She let him use her phone to call his father and girlfriend, after which he began crying. That was the beginning of establishing trust.

Taisha and the team hadn't known him for long, but because the COVID numbers were exceptionally high, his family wasn't allowed to be in the ED. He felt even more alone and isolated, but he was thankful that our team was able to wait with him before he went upstairs. He didn't want to go to the OR, but Taisha convinced him to go. Because of the relationship that he was developing with Taisha, the surgeons allowed her to go with him to the pre-op area, waiting with him before the surgery; fortunately, it was successful.

During Javaun's week-long hospitalization, Taisha saw him regularly, along with some of the intervention team members. He was kind of standoffish on the initial encounter because the team had on their KAVI T-shirts and he worried they were "the cops." He asked a lot of questions: Who are you? What do you do? Why are you seeing me?

While hospitalized, Javaun was cared for by the trauma surgeons who operated on him, the hospital social workers, and the KAVI team. He still wasn't able to see his family while in the hospital and recovering from his surgery, but the KAVI team was able to see him daily. They would visit him for anywhere from a few minutes to a couple of hours throughout the day, continuing to build their bond.

Our violence intervention specialists provided emotional support and served as liaisons between social workers, surgeons, and Javaun. Because he was uninsured and his green card was expired, he was set up for Emergency Medicaid, which in New York State is designed to help temporary and undocumented immigrants pay for their emergency medical care. While healing from his injuries, he was seen daily by Taisha, Bennie, and Natasha, KAVI's case manager, who helped coordinate pending outpatient services and a safe haven for him once he was discharged from the hospital so he would be protected from the guys who stabbed him. The team's job was to make sure Javaun would be OK once he was out, but also to be sure he wouldn't seek revenge.

Javaun had been born in Jamaica but came to New York City with his father and stepmother when he was around eight or nine years old. He wasn't close to his biological mother, as she was addicted to drugs during his early years and left him and his father before he was two years old. (He wouldn't see her again until he was fif-teen.) At age thirteen he was already throwing up gang signs and was being recruited by the Bloods gang in his home neighborhood of Brownsville. Going to high school was more of a formality but helped get him further into gang life. Looking for a family beyond his own, he joined the Bloods. It gave him a level of protection, but the consequences of his affiliation exceeded the support he was given. And being part of the Bloods was undoubtedly an ed-ucation in using violence as a way of getting what you needed and wanted. He transferred to a new school his sophomore year and during the first week there he was jumped by Crips. Going to school didn't prove to be safe for him. More than 80 percent of the people he knew at school were in gangs, he told me. After going to more than twenty different suspension school sites around the city, he dropped out to spend more time in the streets.

Before the age of twenty-one he had multiple gun possession charges, with the latest landing him in prison for more than two years. The only positive thing that came out of prison was that he completed his GED.

After he was discharged from the hospital, Javaun was seen weekly by KAVI intervention specialists, who sometimes spoke to him daily. They offered to accompany him from his home to the hospital during his appointments, and he gladly accepted. He was scared of being reinjured and worried about his "opps," or opposition, his enemies coming around to find him while he was vulnerable.

Since our first encounter with him, he has distanced himself from some of the Bloods to help remain safe and away from sit-uations that might get him in jail, injured again, or even killed. Bennie personally raised money for him to renew his green card, which had expired during the COVID pandemic. His application was recently approved. The team provided job placement assis-tance to help secure full-time employment. The best part of the story is that Javaun is now a full-time employee at Kings County Hospital doing patient transportation. He is actively applying to college, and working part-time with KAVI, co-facilitating group workshops with other violent-trauma victim survivors.

COVID impacted KAVI's programs, as it did everything and everyone around the planet. Wingate High School (one of the sites for KAVI's school program) and Kings County Hospital are both located in East Flatbush, a neighborhood in New York City that was hit hard during the pandemic, with disruption, death, and sorrow everywhere. Given the added chaos of school closings and off-and-on remote schooling, it was nearly impossible to provide consistent school intervention services and maintain the delicate, vital relationships we'd been building with student participants, their families, and their teachers. There was heartbreak all around and we had our share, personally and professionally.

Pre-COVID, KAVI worked in person with about 250 high school and middle school kids. Unsurprisingly, that number was decimated during the pandemic. But we're rebuilding now and restructuring. We have more staff and finally have a data analyst so we can track what we're doing. We currently have 170 students and are in the process of expanding programs to other schools around New York City.

Since the start of our first KAVI school group in 2011, the population we're working with has expanded a bit. We still work with kids who have been getting into fights and have some gang involvement and affiliations. Some kids have been mandated by the school to participate in KAVI as part of their in-school probation or in-school suspension; many others have self-selected to come and participate. There is a misconception that every kid we work with has been involved in gang activity or has a history of being violent. Some have done well in school and have never been in a physical fight, but they see violence in their communities and have developed anxiety, internalizing the stress from their environment. We've had kids who were at the top of their class, but because they witnessed murders or were exposed to extensive amounts of violence in the home or neighborhood, they have had a hard time coping. Some of them stopped doing well in school, had difficulty sleeping, and suffered from depression. The KAVI circle has become a safe space for comradery and for processing the trauma they have experienced. If someone needs more support than our circles can offer, we have licensed mental health practitioners who we recommend to them. We're seeing the effects of trauma outside of school, with kids seeking out KAVI because of the safe space we offer.

Our facilitators had traditionally been a combination of teaching artists, doctors, medical and public health students, professional mediators, and community organizers. We still use some of them as facilitators, but borrowing from accepted interventions addressing HIV, the majority of our facilitators are now peer facilitators, rather than more established professionals. The peer facilitators are a little older than the participants but closer in age than our original facilitators, making them a little easier to relate to socially, but just as effective. Some of our peers are former KAVI program participants and work with us as paid staff members; others volunteer as a way to pay forward what they learned personally and with KAVI. Our mission is best summed up in this statement from our literature.

The classrooms, hallways, cafeterias, and gyms of our schools should be safe sanctuaries for our young people—free of the violence and conflicts on the streets of our communities. They should be safe spaces where young people learn, grow, socialize, thrive, and come into their own as happy adults—and should leave with a sense of accomplishment, clearly focused on building lives of successful families, careers and fulfilment.

The reality is that young people often bring conflicts and social/emotional concerns from their homes and communities into school with them.

Helping our students and schools create a safe and nurturing learning environment goes beyond academics and acquiring skills. It includes the tools and strategies to be able engage in productive relationships with teachers, staff, and other authorities, peers, mentors, and friends.

To help create this nurturing environment and in response to the high numbers of youth being seen for intentional injuries in the KCHC Emergency Department, KAVI offers violence prevention and intervention programs and curriculum in local high schools.

All young people in the schools where we work are invited to participate in KAVI Queens, KAVI Kings and KAVI Royalty, though we focus our programming on youth directly impacted by violence or who may be at risk of being impacted by violence. Many of the youth have revealed dangerous behaviors and the likelihood for engaging in future violent activity. Therefore, KAVI's prevention services in the schools include workshops for "safe spaces" to talk about the issues and influences that led to violence and to consider alternatives.

Our school-based program includes a 32-week module, group-level intervention that takes a deep look at the many ways that youth were experiencing violence through race, gender, and other structural issues. This led to the inclusion of training modules on racial and social justice, restorative justice, and trauma-informed care to address the deeper psychosocial impacts of violence with our youth to our curriculum. KAVI students now have parallel school-based youth programs—one for young men (KAVI Kings) and one for young women (KAVI Queens), and one for students who identify as LGBTQIA+ and their allies (KAVI Royalty).

KAVI Royalty is a co-ed group of students that currently meets at HSPS (High School for Public Service) every Wednesday afternoon. This is an extremely dynamic and creative group. A good number (but not all) of Royalty participants identify as LGBTQIA+. Some students have discussed the difficulties they are experiencing at home and in the community because of their sexuality and how they identify. For example, the majority of KAVI Royalty's participants come from conservative households where being openly gay or gender-nonconforming, or exploring sexuality, is not permitted. The rise in young people identifying as LGBTQIA+ in our schools is significant, making the Royalty group even more important for creating an additional safe space for them to help the trauma that many of them have experienced.

The focus is to enable participants achieve their potential, strengthen their sense of self and handle conflict more readily so they can do better in school, succeed in their careers, and create lasting positive change in their communities.

Our programs, provided through the school year, our peer facilitators and coordinator help our student to . . .

- Get the support they need to succeed in school.
- Make better choices in their relationships with friends and family to be able to stay safe and walk away from violence.
- Access a more supportive school environment that offers opportunities to encourage their passions, dreams, and careers.

Our curriculum uses a group-based learning approach where young people learn from each other's experiences and problem solve together to overcome challenges, handle difficult social and family situations, and take steps to realize their dreams and passions.

Our skilled peer facilitators come from the neighborhoods where our young people live. We strongly believe that solutions to public safety and violence come directly from the communities most impacted. Young people involved in our programming may later become on-staff peer facilitators themselves.

We integrate restorative justice practices to hold young people accountable for their actions while keeping them in community and helping them heal.

We believe restorative justice practices are an important part of building a more supportive school environment. KAVI team members advocate on behalf of young people to school staff, in disciplinary meetings and with parents.

DANNY

"I think I want to be a photographer, Mr. Russell," said Danny, flipping through the pages. He was fourteen, bright, with a wild afro. Russell Frederick, one of KAVI's newer facilitators and a professional photographer was helping run the workshop. (Russell is now one of KAVI's board members.) It was early 2012 and for the past few months a group of young men from the High School for Public Service (HSPS) and the School for International Arts and

Business had been meeting for a few hours on Friday mornings. Most recently they were studying photographs and magazines in the first workshop we developed for KAVI, called Positive Images, a twelve-week exploration of race, gender, and leadership through photography and film. Many students were randomly flipping through the pages, but a few, Danny in particular, became en- grossed with images, devouring the magazines with a laser focus, shutting out the outside world and escaping into another.

I had a special love of photography and pictures, old or recent, and an even greater appreciation of the stories behind those im- ages. It was my hope to share that with the students. As a kid, I would regularly absorb the images found in old family photo albums, memorizing the faces and imagining the events taking place in the background. Whenever my father brought home the envelopes of his freshly developed pictures, I would look at the images for hours, refamiliarizing myself with the people and the activities taking place. I remember an adult telling me that I had a photographic memory, but I don't think that was the case. As with any practice, to quote my mentor and advisor, the late Dean Thomas Blocker, "repetition breeds familiarity." However, looking at images over and over again in real time was leaving in my mind an imprint of the people and an ability to recall names, scenes, and feelings that were going on in them for years to come.

"If you're interested in learning how to take pictures and be a photographer, then let's see about getting you into a class," said Russell. "I'll reach out to the people at the ICP [International Cen- ter of Photography] to see if we can get you into one of their sum- mer courses," he added.

Bayeté, now facilitating groups with KAVI, taught photogra- phy at ICP and NYU. He was excited about the possibility of hav- ing one of our kids spend time exploring creative outlets outside of Brooklyn, an opportunity not often available to less affluent kids, unless they were part of an elite magnet school. Danny lit up at the possibility of taking a course in photography.

When he was alert and engaged, Danny was a good student. However, as likeable and intelligent as he was, he would disappear for a few days at a time. He didn't have a physical illness but dealt with a lot of stress. "I have a lot going on at home and sometimes I gotta smoke and be alone but I don't wanna come to school when I'm like that," he explained to me once. He only wanted to be around if he could be fully present and able to pay attention. One of his teachers, knowing that he'd been part of KAVI, approached me and said, "You should talk to him because he's not doing anything in my class and being lazy." She didn't say that she'd noticed he'd been depressed, excessively sleepy, withdrawn, or even "something was wrong with him, but I don't know how to describe it." The adjective she used to describe him was *lazy*.

The word *lazy* is triggering, but especially when I hear it being used to describe Black kids—and even worse when it comes from a white teacher. My father told me that when he was a kid, one of the biggest ways to insult a person was to tell them their kid was "lazy." There had been a series of caricatures depicting the "lazy Negro" like "Little Sambo" with his exaggerated facial features, lying down eating watermelon, only good for eating and sleeping. When I heard the term, it made me think of those images; whites, often those in power, used the word to describe Blacks working for them doing manual labor. As long as the Negro produced, then they were good; if they didn't produce in a way the white person in power wanted, they became "lazy."

Danny lived in Brownsville, a neighborhood historically known for being rough. I know a lot of great people from Brownsville and they all possess a unique grittiness. Danny possessed that same grit, maybe because he understood the need to survive. More recently, Brownsville was Blood territory, and because of where he lived and the need to ensure his own safety, he became a Blood at fourteen years old.

He had no interest in causing harm to anyone with his relatively new membership, but his survival was based on his ability to navigate safely through his own neighborhood. As protected as he hoped to be with his affiliation, safety wasn't always promised and neither was emotional support. One day, the school's social worker, Ms. Rachel, who referred Danny to KAVI mainly because she'd known of his gang affiliation, called me. "There is something going on personally with Danny. It might be helpful for you to talk to him," she said.

I found Danny, sitting adjacent to the principal's office, in tears. "Dr. Gore, Mr. Russell, I don't know what to do. I'm mad, and I'm upset with what's going on at home. My stepdad beats my mom, in the middle of the night, in front of me and my little sisters. I'm having trouble sleeping. I wanna hurt him. I wanna call the police, but if I do that, then my sisters grow up in a household without a father, just like I did."

Every accumulating strain and stressor have the ability to compromise an individual's physical and mental well-being. These strains are exacerbated dramatically if a person already has a pre-existing mental health challenge like depression, bipolar disorder, schizophrenia, or oppositional defiant disorder, to name a few. I knew Danny had undiagnosed depression based on our conversations and I worried for his safety at home and in the streets.

He watched his mother repeatedly brutalized in his own home. How do you sleep at night if your family's safety is in jeopardy? How are you expected to do well in algebra and to pay attention in English or health class? How is getting a formal education supposed to help you if you are unable to think past survival?

Despite his home life challenges, Danny continued to come to school and the KAVI sessions. His focus began to increase and he seemed less depressed as time passed. Our team made sure he had as much support as we could provide.

Later that spring Danny enrolled in a special youth photography program sponsored by the ICP. He learned how to take pictures with an SLR camera alongside other high school students from around the city. He spent time learning about lighting and exploring how to capture images. He even learned about developing photographs in a dark room the old-fashioned way. He was becoming the artist he wanted to become. One of the shining moments for us was to see him showcase his photographs in an art show. He was proud of what he had created and we were even prouder.

It was inspiring to watch Danny evolve over the course of that year. He opened up more. He came to school more consistently. He displayed levels of vulnerability beyond what we imagined possible, just by telling us intimate details of his personal and home life. He did the hard work. We just helped build a space that allowed him to express himself.

We lost touch with Danny at the end of the summer after his freshman year of high school. He transferred schools and moved out of Brooklyn. I wish he would have stayed with us in KAVI longer but more for my own selfish reasons. Danny was a natural leader. Other students gravitated to him. He wasn't pompous and didn't show a lot of bravado, despite his gang affiliation. The guys in his grade looked up to him. When they saw him coming to our sessions, they also decided it was cool for them to come to the sessions. If they were joking around in workshops and Danny was serious about participating, he sometimes glanced over at them and they would gradually calm down and get more serious. I recently had the good luck to reconnect with Danny after ten years. He's no longer in a gang and is working in retail, where he developed a clothing line, and is raising his infant daughter. He still remembers his time with KAVI in high school and is thankful that our team cared enough to support and advocate on his behalf, something he has taken to heart as a new parent.

ZANE

Zane's story is a great example of how KAVI works in real time. This happened not long after Willis was killed, but this time, KAVI was able to head off the worst. Zane was a student in one of our programs in East Flatbush. He was a likable kid, usually joking around and friendly with staffers and other students. He had a lot of promise and potential, but like a lot of KAVI kids, a lot to overcome. He was born in Guyana, and since his arrival in the US as a toddler, he and his family had lived in East New York, an underdeveloped and underfunded tough neighborhood in Brooklyn. "The first time I saw someone killed was when I was about three or four years old," he said early on in our time together at KAVI. "A neighbor walking close to our house was robbed by some guys and had his throat cut by a machete."

By the time he was a teenager, Zane had witnessed much more death and violence firsthand and had been to more than thirty funerals of friends and family members. He had proudly claimed being a member of the Bloods since he was in elementary school. Some of the members of his family were Bloods, and being a Blood meant having a family beyond a family, having a true sense of protection on the streets, and not having to walk around in fear. By the time I met Zane, he'd developed a routine of carrying a gun or a knife most of the time but leaving both at a friend's house in order to avoid the school's metal detectors.

He'd gotten into a bunch of fights in school and had been suspended quite a few times for fighting or cursing out teachers. But if you were on his good side, you would never believe such behavior was possible from him. He brought life to every meeting.

That's why it was especially noticeable to me one day in a KAVI meeting when Zane was far off, his face set in a frown, his eyes narrowed, staring angrily at one specific fellow student. I understood why Zane might be angry with this guy. The guy had his own set of personal challenges but could be obnoxious at times and say unwarranted things for attention. I figured he probably said something silly or highly annoying earlier in the day. But I was concerned about the level of anger on Zane's face.

Zane and I had always gotten along, and he showed the utmost respect to me and the other male facilitators. "We will advocate for you as long as you keep it a hunnid," Russell Frederick, our program director, had told him and all the young people in the program. ("Hunnid" was short for "hundred" and slang for being 100 percent honest.) So long as a student in KAVI is 100 percent honest and 100 percent real when meeting with us, we will support them in whatever way possible. We came with enough knowledge and enough shared experience that we could be real with them too. Being mindful and present is the simplest way to honor your comrades, regardless of circumstance, and that code has been central to our success at KAVI.

With that in mind, I tapped him on the shoulder and signaled for him to leave the table. There were no "oohs" or "ahhs" from the rest of the group because everyone got pulled from the table at some point to talk outside.

Without even my prompting, Zane kept it a hunnid immediately. He calmly said that his fellow student was going to "get what's coming to him. He won't be a problem for anyone after this afternoon." Whoa. This was far more serious than I had anticipated. I signaled to my fellow facilitators to come join me and we found an unoccupied conference room nearby.

"What do you mean, 'You won't have to worry about him by this afternoon'?" I said.

"I put a hit out on him," he replied, with little sign of remorse. Dr. Ramon Gist, a fellow physician and pediatric intensivist (currently KAVI's clinical director), Russell, and I were briefly stunned into silence.

What would make a teenager put a hit out on another person, especially another teenager? I couldn't wrap my head around what could be so serious that he wanted someone's life to be taken away. In all honesty, I don't think Zane fully understood the gravity of the action, either. His decision to put a hit out was an almost automated response because he had been trained to retaliate when he felt disrespected or angry. What caused this homicidal rage?

"He kept talking shit. . . . He disrespected me. . . . He plays too much." He wasn't even able to articulate a specific offense. But he'd been "dissed" and that was enough. Being disrespected meant that a boundary had been violated. For a lot of the kids we work with, disrespect, whether actual or perceived, is grounds for fighting or, as in Zane's case, even worse.

Disrespect came in many forms, including someone dating a person you recently dated and being made fun of in public, like in school or online in a social media post. It could be that someone was "talking bad" about your mother or grandmother (I seldom, if ever, heard about fights started because of a person making fun of someone's father), or dishonoring something that you held sacred, like your family, your gang, or even the block you lived on; all were used as ample pretext for violence.

The situation was a first for me. Should I call the police and file a report? If I did, one life could be saved, but another one would end, for all intents and purposes. Zane might have been arrested and gone to jail, ending what remained of his adolescence and his life as he knew it. I was equally scared that three people would lose their lives—the target, the person who pulled the trigger, and the one who ordered the hit. Their families would be left behind to pick up the pieces.

We continued to talk to Zane and listen closely to his pain and anger, allowing him to find the presence of mind on his own to change the outcome of his most recent act of anger. Calmly, we asked him pointed questions that began to make an impact, bit by bit:

What are you going to do if other people make you mad?
Are you going to put a hit out on them too?
What happens if you get caught?
You ready to go to prison?
You really 'bout that life?
What else do you have to live for?

He got quiet and more pensive. "What about Moms and your sister?" I'd spoken to his mother a few times and knew how close they were. Also, his sister was pregnant, and he was about to become a new uncle.

We sat around the table for about an hour talking with him in a way I imagine elders might have in the past. Finally, without us asking directly, he took out his phone and called off the hit. A few years later, when I talked to him about the incident, he didn't even remember why he'd set it up. We had helped him see his way clear of a dangerous impulse, to step away from the hair trigger. But it remains both a triumph and a clear reminder of how easy it is for anyone, even a kid like Zane, to unleash unthinkable violence, and why it's so important that we do everything we can to prevent it.

Zane graduated from high school more than five years ago and has completely distanced himself from his gang days. He is now working full-time for UPS and helps raise his niece and nephew.

Some of the most challenging kids we work with at KAVI, and a significant number of the patients I've treated in the ED, seem to confine their emotional lives to either happiness or anger. They haven't learned to manage or name any other feelings.

But the emotion I see the most in my work is anger, often followed by lashing out. The norm of the community—the one we and other organizations are working to change—is that lashing out and retaliation are the ways to solve problems and conflicts. Being "respected" is the most important thing for these emerging adults, and they do what they think they have to do in order to get their version of that. Also, often, the cycle of violence is perpetuated by a trauma that is unacknowledged and unmanaged. It puts you on a hair trigger, the kind Zane was living on, so that simple annoyance is an emotion to be answered by murder.

The problem in the traumatized mind is that anything that isn't happiness is considered anger. Feelings of disgust or fear become anger, so do feelings of shame, envy, anxiety, and awkwardness; without reflection, these emotions all tend to roll up on one another and become one furious mess in the mind of a trauma victim.

For exactly this reason, there were regular conversations with our students, particularly the guys, about understanding their emotions and consequences to behavior.

As we tried to talk Zane down, I thought, too, of what an enormous loss Willis's murder, less than a year before, had been for us all. I thought about what he would've said to Zane. They were both members of the Bloods, and because of the gang relationship they'd had a special bond. One of the reasons Zane came to our sessions so regularly was because Willis was there. "Young told me it's not what you walk away from, but what you walk away with," he recalled. In that moment, I felt Willis's spirit with us all.

CHAPTER 14

IN HONOR OF WILLIS

EVERYBODY IS GOOD until they're not.

I had been working in emergency medicine for more than ten years when Willis was killed. Death and tragedy were a regular part of life. And I thought I was "good." Much like many of our patients after trauma, I tried to keep moving forward without a minute's pause or break. I even worked in the critical care and trauma area of the emergency department the night of his funeral, seeing patients in the very same place he was brought to after being stabbed multiple times before his untimely death.

During that shift, as happens so often, we treated a patient who was the victim of violence. The patient had arrived shortly before I came to work. He'd been shot multiple times in his extremities and was in serious but stable condition and not likely to die immediately without being treated. Before I walked into the room to see him, one of the nurses alerted me about his background. I'd met him before. He and I had met because I pronounced his little brother dead a few years prior after he was shot and killed by the police. Another senseless shooting—two in one family.

After going in and out of the patient's room checking on him, reassessing his condition and giving him updates on his diagnostic studies, his mother entered the room and recognized me immediately. It was more than awkward because after recognizing me, she spoke to me, asking questions about her son's condition just like any caring parent; however, she stopped looking at me directly. She looked at the nurses and made eye contact with them but continued to avoid looking at me when she asked me additional questions. I knew the avoidance of eye contact was her not wanting to be triggered or reminded of the circumstances in which we first met, since I was the one who gave her the news that her younger son had been killed. I, too, felt uneasy and didn't want to go in the room to answer her questions because it was triggering for me. I entered the room one last time to let the patient and family know that he was going to be admitted for further observation and monitoring, to which he agreed. His mother then shouted out, looking me in the eyes with tears streaming down her face, "Did my other son say anything to you before he died?" I began to tremble immediately after hearing her words, but I couldn't answer because he did say something to me. His last comprehendible words were "Don't let me die," shortly before he lost his vital signs and died in the trauma bay. I just told the mother, "I'm sorry," while fighting back my own tears, and ran out of the room into the bathroom to breathe. I melted down in the bathroom and had an uncontrollable cry and was breathing fast and had dry heaves with hiccups. It took about ten minutes for me to pull myself together so I could get back to the CCT and finish seeing patients for the remaining five and half hours of my shift. I put on my glasses to help mask my red eyes and walked around a lot so my coworkers couldn't see I was hurting or trembling. When I sat still at the computer terminal to write notes, I just tensed up my muscles so that people couldn't see me shaking. No one asked me if I was alright, but I didn't tell them either. It was OK for doctors to not feel well, but there was an unwritten rule that we had to get our emotions in check so we could continue to work—I could be emotional after work but not during. There was just the expectation that I continue to work as usual. Do you think I was providing quality care? I knew I wasn't—my ability to do so had been compromised by my own exhaustion and culminating grief.

A few days later, the first signs that I was having a problem appeared. They were initially very subtle—the sounds and smells of the ED seemed more annoying than usual. But I chalked it up to fatigue. Then later, my hands would tingle whenever I walked into the hospital, and the tingling increased when I went into the ED to work. I found it more difficult to talk to patients and coworkers. Sometimes, out of the blue, I'd have these episodes of rapid breathing. Other times, I had the shakes.

I realized that I was having panic attacks, and it scared the shit out of me. It had never happened to me before. I was supposed to taking care of other people, but the truth is, I wasn't taking good care of myself. The thing that freaked me out the most was not having control of what I was experiencing. What's more, the possibility of a panic attack coming on while I was working made me even more anxious.

I needed to get some help, but like most docs, I avoided going to see a professional—what is it they say? "Physician, heal thyself." I distracted myself with more work. I knew it wouldn't help but I tried that anyway.

I continued my daily meditation, which helped me be able to fall asleep at night. I further immersed myself in my marital arts practice—training and studying Brazilian jiu-jitsu. After training, my body regularly hurt all over. That, combined with intense physical activity and the process of repeatedly practicing a movement that I sucked at, was therapeutic. But it wasn't enough.

Eventually I gave in and went to therapy. I'd gone to therapy before, but really didn't want to return because I didn't feel like having one of those long ugly cries, where everything comes out of your face, and because looking at my patterns of behavior in therapy was embarrassing. The voice of the high school kid inside of me, the one who tried to brush everything off—was still there.

At one point in the session, I got silent when the therapist asked me the simple question, "Why?" While I waited for some kind of insight to pop into my head for why I was feeling the way I was feeling, the therapist told me my problem was empathy.

I kind of looked at her weird, like *huh*? I'd always thought empathy was a good thing. As a doctor it's important to understand and share the feelings of others. Even in med school we were taught that having empathy would help us develop a better understanding of what our patients were going through, to figure out the optimal way to care for them. After further conversation with the therapist, I came to realize my problem wasn't understanding the feelings of others; it was sharing their feelings.

In sharing their feelings, I was taking on the stress and pain of patients, and I was even taking on the stress and pain of friends. It was almost as if I needed to be part of their suffering in order to find a bond with them. What I needed to learn to do—what I have done over time, which KAVI has helped me with—is to detach with love. My other realization was that I wasn't giving myself any room to truly grieve Willis's death. That day in the therapist's office ended up being one of the most significant of my medical career. She helped me begin to see how to avoid burning out, how to keep on going, how to continue caring about, but not drowning in, the lives of my patients. And she helped me see that I had to take the time in my heart to mourn Willis. The only way to keep our work going was to mourn the loss and then celebrate the life by saving others.

The United States is perhaps the most violent of the developed nations. While my experience with treating violence has been entirely in predominantly Black, Brown, and urban neighborhoods, the violence spans coast to coast, across all ethnicities and within many communities. At KAVI, we'll continue to do our part. I'm proud of what we've done so far. We have students who are in college, and one student from our first group is in medical school at Brown. We have students at my alma mater, Morehouse. We've been around long enough now that we have employees who are former participants, and they're doing everything from facilitating school-based workshops to working with our hospital-based intervention program. I talked with my parents, who grew up during the civil rights era of the 1960s (remember my dad was a member of SCLC with Dr. Martin Luther King Jr.), and the one thing that they articulated about these organizations, which doesn't always happen, is that people need to make sure they pass on that torch and prepare for succession. There must be leaders in waiting who can run the organization when the time comes; otherwise, these great ideas and their impact wind up dying with the founders. For my entire career—premed, med student, resident, attending physician, and right up through the founding of MMSEM, KAVI, and beyond—I've always made sure that mentoring was an integral part of what I do. Now in its fourteenth year, MMSEM counts among its leaders some of the folks who participated in the program. If you train people to lead, then they're in the position to deeply affect their communities in years to come.

KAVI is a dynamic organization that has to keep changing. It has to respond to public health disasters like COVID, of course, but there are also other considerations. When we first started in 2009, social media existed but was in no way the pervasive force it is now. Instagram didn't exist, there was no Snapchat or TikTok, people weren't using Facebook to gangbang and put out threats. By the time this book is published, the evolving digital space will create even more invasive social changes. So now KAVI works with our team members to make sure that they understand social media and that they talk to the patients and students we work with about how social media can be a tool for good or be another kind of weapon. Like coastal palm trees, if you can be flexible, you will survive the storm, but if you're too rigid and have an unwillingness to bend, if you're unable to adapt, you'll break.

We are expanding our reach and taking on more school sites. Right now we see patients in the emergency department and trauma clinic and in our work with schools, but we are trying to increase access for patients at all clinics and at any point of entry. We are also working to provide follow-up and follow-through for patients, to increase our own training, and to educate more volunteers and more physicians on a larger scale. I do hope that one day our services will no longer be needed and have a goal for us to become obsolete. In honor of Willis, I'll never lose sight of that goal.

Just as important, we will continue working with other organizations across the country to make sure that the models of violence intervention and prevention become part of hospital protocols and school curriculum everywhere. Because of my work abroad,

I even envision the models of organizations like KAVI spreading internationally.

The mission begins with the recognition that violence is a public health problem that needs to be treated as one in order to be cured. We need to understand, at a most basic level, that treating this disease needs to be a priority for our government, medical, mental health, and social welfare sectors. We need to redefine how great the potential is to save lives, not just of victims, but of their families and communities. Treating epidemics like this requires significant investments and resources so we can understand the roots of violence, including causes like poverty, lack of opportunity, underinvestment in communities of color and immigrant communities, and under-resourced schools, community centers, and hospitals. And we need to treat those root causes and implement policies to ensure the treatments become law, with an ability to mitigate future violent events.

It shouldn't take years to get adequate financial support for anti-violence and community development programs. Nor should it take years to federally regulate gun access and ban assault weapons. This is an investment in human well-being. Cities, municipalities, states, and the federal government need to seek ways to stem this epidemic from within the affected communities, especially by engaging the people most impacted by this issue, just as they did with COVID. We know that easy accessibility of weapons impacts the rate of homicides, which is why the US homicide rate is seven times higher than that of other affluent nations, and our firearm homicide rate is 25.2 times higher than other high-income countries.[1] We know that quality social relationships have a positive benefit on a person's health.[2] We know that early detection of a disease can help contain it and prevent it from spreading.[3] We know that supportive spaces have a nurturing effect on community development and individual well-being.[4]

The long-term solution to the problems of violence has to be greater than a vaccine. We work to prevent untimely death, but we need to go further by supporting a high-quality and sustainable life. The final goal is not the mere absence of trauma and violence but the promotion of well-being for the individual and their community.

It is beyond understandable to ask repeatedly why these conditions of human conflict, which result in the loss of life, continue to exist. More questions emerge when trying to figure out what to do to fix the problems, but the answers aren't that difficult to find. As is most often the case, the answers lie within the communities, among the grassroots and the people themselves. I hope that, with vision and resources, organizations like KAVI and those I describe in the resource section—those based in various parts of the country and those that have yet to be developed—will be able to pivot from primarily treating the effects of violence to working to prevent violence and trauma entirely. I hope you will join me in this work.

RESOURCES FOR VIOLENCE PREVENTION AND TREATMENT

THE GOOD NEWS IS that programs like KAVI work. In general, the implementation of preventive health measures helps to decrease the development of chronic healthcare issues that impact longevity and quality of life.[1] Education on health and early detection is cheaper than treating full-blown medical problems. Violence is no exception. One of the biggest risk factors for violent injury is a previous violent injury. Violence intervention programs have been shown to decrease recurrent violent injuries, which means lower costs for rehospitalizations. Compared to hospitals without intervention programs, those hospitals that do have them have demonstrated the ability to increase life expectancy and quality of life.[2]

I hope KAVI can continue to grow and also serve as a model for other organizations all over the nation and, eventually, across the globe. Here are some organizations that I am especially indebted to and appreciative of for their support, guidance, and collaboration.

MAN UP! INC.

Man Up! Inc., a community-based nonprofit dedicated to providing services for neighborhood improvement was borne out of the concerns of Black men in the East New York section of Brooklyn.

Some of their services include violence intervention and interruption, as well as youth programming and job training. Man Up! Inc.'s violence intervention uses the Cure Violence model and is a part of the Cure Violence coalition of violence prevention programs. Man Up! Inc. and SOS were KAVI's first community partners in providing violence prevention services at Kings County Hospital. The founder of Man Up! Inc. is Brother A. T. Mitchell, whom Mayor Eric Adams named New York City's czar for the Gun Violence Prevention Task Force. See manupinc.org for more information.

SAVE OUR STREETS

Save Our Streets (SOS) is a program under the Center for Court Innovation, dedicated to ending "gun violence at the neighborhood level by changing local norms around violence and creating opportunities for meaningful educational and employment opportunities within the community." SOS was one of KAVI's first hospital program partners. Their expertise and insight have helped shift violence intervention around New York City. The Center for Court Innovation was created in 1993 to address low-level offending around Times Square; the project's success in reducing both crime and incarceration led the New York State Unified Court System to partner with the Fund for the City of New York to establish the Center for Court Innovation as an independent nonprofit dedicated to justice reform. For more information, see www.innovatingjustice.org/programs/save-our-streets-sos.

CURE VIOLENCE

Cure Violence (formerly CeaseFire) is a global violence intervention and prevention program founded by fellow physician, epidemiologist, and former head of WHO's Intervention Development Unit Dr. Gary Slutkin. After launching in the West Garfield Park neighborhood of Chicago in the early 2000s, an area with a high rate of violent trauma, there was a reduction in shootings of 67 percent in the first year in that community. These efforts are largely attributed to the dedicated and intense work by the Cure Violence team. The success of Cure Violence has been felt around the US and even across the world; programs using the Cure Violence model are being used in Baltimore, New York City, New Orleans, Puerto Rico, Colombia, Jamaica, and elsewhere. In addition to running their programs, Cure Violence has been training countless others in their methods and in violence prevention across the globe. For more information, see cvg.org.

YOUTH ALIVE!

Established in 1991, Youth ALIVE! is a nonprofit organization based in Oakland, California. They founded the first hospital-based violence intervention program, called Caught in the Crossfire (CiC), which serves trauma centers in Alameda County, California. CiC was the model for KAVI's hospital intervention, since we believed in their philosophy: "Where there is violence, there can be healing." Youth ALIVE's programs have been highly successful, engaging people who have been injured due to violence, or who are at risk for engaging in violence, and meeting with them on the streets, in schools, in homes, and at hospital bedsides. Their services include advocacy work, violence interruption and prevention, relationship building, and case management through a team of highly skilled and trained credible messengers and community members. For more information, see YouthAlive.org.

VIOLENCE INTERVENTION PROGRAM

Violence Intervention Program (VIP) in Baltimore is an evidence-based program started by Dr. Carnell Cooper at the University of Maryland Medical Center. Dr. Cooper started VIP in response to seeing victims of traumatic violent injuries be readmitted to the hospital for subsequent and often more violent injuries. In Baltimore, violence is the leading cause of death for young adults and is widely recognized as a public health issue. For more information, see umms.org/ummc/health-services/shock-trauma/center-injury-prevention-policy/violence/intervention-program.

VIOLENCE INTERVENTION
AND ADVOCACY PROGRAM

The Violence Intervention and Advocacy Program (VIAP) was started in 2006 by Dr. Thea James with support from Dr. Ed Bernstein. The program provides comprehensive violence intervention and prevention wraparound services at Boston Medical Center and additional sites serving the Greater Boston community and the state of Massachusetts. Coincidentally, Dr. James gave me my earliest exposure to emergency medicine when I was an undergraduate student back in 1996. VIAP provided early mentorship and support to help develop KAVI and trained the early group of KAVI's hospital intervention team. Dr. James and VIAP are founding partners of the National Network for Hospital-Based Violence Intervention Programs, which is now known as the Health Alliance for Violence Intervention. For more information, see bmc.org/violence-intervention-advocacy-program.

HEALING HURT PEOPLE

Healing Hurt People (HHP) is violence intervention and prevention program based in Philadelphia, with programs also in Portland, Oregon, and Chicago. Prior to launching KAVI's programming, I studied the work of Dr. John Rich, a primary care physician and public health expert, who was one of the first people I ever heard speak about violence as a public health issue. Years later, I would have the pleasure of meeting and learning from the core HHP team and its other founding members, including Dr. Rich; Dr. Ted Corbin, an emergency physician; Linda Rich, a psychotherapist with extensive experience in health policy and program planning; and Dr. Sandra Bloom, a psychiatrist who developed the Sanctuary Model. The Sanctuary Model is an evidence-based template and a set of tools used to help effectively recognize, understand, and serve the needs of people having a traumatic experience and the organizations working with them. HHP has gained significant national attention and is a leader in the movement to end violence using a public health approach. For more information, see drexel.edu/cnsj/healing-hurt-people /overview.

THE FORTUNE SOCIETY

The Fortune Society, based in New York City, provides support services for people returning home after being incarcerated. Formerly incarcerated individuals have a plethora of challenges to overcome adjusting to a new life. The Fortune Society has been critical in helping provide and coordinate support for education, affordable housing, substance abuse treatment, health care, job training, and family services. We at KAVI have been referring clients in need of services to the Fortune Society for years. We now have a linkage program with them, where some of their former clients are working with KAVI providing violence intervention services in the hospital. For more information, see fortunesoci ety.org.

SAFE HORIZON

Established in 1978, Safe Horizon is one of the oldest victim assistance programs in New York City. It provides support for families and traumatized individuals who have experienced partner violence, sexual violence, human trafficking, child abuse, houselessness, and more. Their services include crime victim assistance, help engaging with law enforcement and filing police reports, legal support for both family and criminal court, and counseling services, to name a few. KAVI has been partnering and working with Safe Horizon for a number of years, utilizing their resources, making referrals, and working with some of their team members in our hospital intervention program. For more information, see safehorizon.org.

MAYOR'S OFFICE OF CRIMINAL JUSTICE

The Mayor's Office of Criminal Justice (MOCJ) was created to help provide guidance to the New York City's mayor's office on policies and issues related to criminal justice and the maintenance and "improvement of a fair and equitable justice system." MOCJ has been instrumental in bringing together community stakeholders, institutions, and concerned citizens, providing strategic development to decrease rates of incarceration, unnecessary arrests, recidivism, and ultimately to ensure the well-being of New

York City. MOCJ has also been a key supporter in securing resources that have allowed KAVI, as well as many other violence prevention organizations around the city, to operate and grow. For more information, see criminaljustice.cityofnewyork.us.

GANGSTAS MAKING ASTRONOMICAL COMMUNITY CHANGES

Gangstas Making Astronomical Community Changes (G-MACC) is a Brooklyn-based violence intervention program within New York City's Cure Violence Crisis Management System. The organization was founded by Brooklynite youth advocate and national gang specialist Mr. Shanduke McPhatter as a way to help disrupt cycles of violence and incarceration through community development. The program's vision "is based upon changing the lives of those caught in the street life, which involves drugs, guns, violence, prison and the overall gangsta mentality," according to its website. In addition to providing street outreach and violence interruption services in the East Flatbush and Fort Greene sections of Brooklyn and programs on Rikers Island prison, G-MACC members work alongside KAVI, providing violence intervention services at Kings County Hospital Center. G-MACC provides resources to youths and adults in and out of the prison system. G-MACC's philosophy is summed up in this website statement: "G-MACC Inc. is committed to making positive change by reaching out to residents of all ages in communities ravaged by gun violence and gang activity. By providing tools and resources to young and old alike, G-MACC helps people reflect, learn, act, and evolve to embrace the healthy, caring, stable individual within, and to transform the surrounding community through positivity and activism." For more information, see gangstamackin.com.

BROOKLYN COMBINE

The Brooklyn Combine is a community organization consisting of artisans, attorneys, and creatives, dedicated to challenging social norms and providing youth leadership development and education initiatives in law, business, and community development.

The Brooklyn Combine is committed to "sustaining the culture that supports and advances the well-being of oppressed peoples in general and the Pan-African diaspora in particular," according to their website. These special friends and comrades of mine—including Dr. Keith White, Esq. (KAVI board member); Kenneth Montgomery, Esq.; Phillip Shung; Mali X; Jazz; and Barnabas Crosby—have cultivated something beyond a think tank to engage disruptive thinkers and doers who have been responsible for helping guide and challenge the social constructs that exist within our borough. I am indebted to their guidance and friendship in this work. For more information, see bklyncombine.com.

ELITE LEARNERS

Founded by Brooklyn activist Ms. Camara Jackson, Elite Learners is a school- and community-based organization based in the Brownsville section of Brooklyn, which provides athletic, educational, and mentorship programming to youths and their families to build community leaders. In addition to providing youth-building programs and support, Elite Learners provides violence intervention and anti–gun violence initiatives in the Brownsville and Flatbush neighborhoods of Brooklyn. For more information, see elitelearners.org.

ACCLIVUS

Acclivus is a community health organization and hospital- and community-based violence intervention program serving the Chicagoland area hospitals, including Advocate Health Care, Advocate Illinois Masonic Medical Center, John H. Stroger Jr. Hospital of Cook County, Mount Sinai Hospital, St. Bernard Hospital, and Northwestern Memorial Hospital. Acclivus provides trauma-informed care, needs assessments, and therapeutic case management services, structured to connect patients with resources that reduce risk of violent reinjury and further involvement in community violence. Their founder and CEO, Mr. LeVon Stone, has been a tremendous force serving the greater Chicago community. I first met Mr. Stone in the early days of KAVI at conferences but later was fortunate to learn more from his expertise while visiting Chicago, which helped shape and morph KAVI's hospital intervention program. For more information, see acclivusinc.org.

GUNS DOWN LIFE UP

Guns Down Life Up (GDLU) is the brainchild of people connector Mr. Joe Schick. Initially it was developed as a social media campaign to increase awareness of gun violence within NYC's Health + Hospitals network system (H+H is the largest network of public hospitals in the US). However, under the marketing genius of Mr. James Dobbins, it morphed into a citywide violence prevention campaign. Seeing a need for more than awareness, GDLU evolved into an intervention program and now provides violence intervention and prevention services, run by Dobbins, at Lincoln Hospital in the South Bronx. GDLU provides youth programming and comprehensive wraparound services for victims and survivors of intentional violence treated at Lincoln Hospital. For more information, see gunsdownlifeup.org.

HEALTH ALLIANCE FOR VIOLENCE INTERVENTION

The Health Alliance for Violence Intervention (HAVI), formerly known as the National Network of Hospital-Based Violence Intervention Programs, is a nationwide organization that "fosters hospital and community collaborations to advance equitable, trauma-informed care and violence intervention and prevention programs," according to its website. The HAVI is made up of multidisciplinary violence intervention experts from local government, private organizations, public health experts, and credible messengers and has been critical to the advancement of trauma-informed care practices around the world, especially within spaces providing medical care to vulnerable populations. Through the HAVI network, and their respective conferences and trainings, organizations from around the world, including KAVI, have been able to enhance their expertise with best practices for violence intervention and prevention. For more information, see thehavi.org.

POP ON VIOLENCE

POP (Protect Outreach and Prevention) on Violence is a youth violence prevention and intervention program based in Merrillville, Indiana, and founded by emergency physician Dr. Michael McGee and trauma surgeon Dr. Reuben Rutland. Recognizing that violence permeates communities well before people become patients, POP on Violence's youth-oriented programs include school-based conflict mediation, a health and law profession enrichment program, career exploration, and Code Blue, a program created to improve relationships with community members, youths, and law enforcement. For more information, see popon violence.org.

TRAUMA RECOVERY AND PREVENTION OF VIOLENCE

Trauma Recovery and Prevention of Violence (TRAP Violence) is a violence prevention program operating under the aegis of the nonprofit MedCEEP, based in Chicago. It was founded by emergency physician Dr. Abdullah Pratt, an attending physician at the University of Chicago Medical Center in the Department of Emergency Medicine, "to educate youth on the structural causes of violence and teach evidence-based approaches to manage conflict with the goal of responding to life stressors by substituting a nonviolent approach." TRAP Violence works with schools and community groups in Chicago and partners with area violence intervention programs Violence Recovery Program and HHP in Chicago. For more information, see medceep.com.

HARLEM MOTHERS SAVE

Out of the trauma of losing two sons to gun violence, Mrs. Jackie Rowe-Adams launched Harlem Mothers SAVE (Stop Another Violent End) to ensure that other families would not lose their loved ones to violence. Harlem Mothers SAVE is one of the older violence intervention programs in New York City. They have been instrumental in galvanizing communities to address gun violence and have been helping lobby for sensible and responsible gun laws both locally and federally. Harlem Mothers SAVE provides summer youth training programs for teens and adolescents, and it provides victims services for individuals and families impacted by gun violence. For more information, see harlemmoth erssave.org.

LIFE CAMP

LIFE Camp (Love Ignites Freedom Through Education Camp) is a community violence intervention program based in Southeast Queens, New York, and is part of New York City's Crisis Management System (CMS). LIFE Camp has combined activism, personal wellness, and crisis management to improve community vitality. These efforts are the result of an incredible team but are largely due to the vision and perseverance of its founder, Erica Ford. Their efforts have created high levels of community support in Southeast Queens, resulting in a record four years without a homicide in their catchment area. Erica's work has benefited communities well beyond Southeast Queens; she has been instrumental in forming CMS, an evidence-based anti–gun violence initiative that amplifies the leadership of community-based solutions to coproduce public safety. She was also a key player in the growth of this pilot, which began with five sites funded at $12 million and evolved into a bureau within the New York City's mayor's office, comprising thirty-four sites throughout the five boroughs, seventeen police precincts, and funding of more than $50 million. For more information, see peaceisalifestyle.com.

67TH PRECINCT CLERGY COUNCIL

Founded by Pastor Gil Monrose, a friend and one of my earliest collaborators in addressing violence in Brooklyn, the 67th Precinct Clergy Council Inc., also known as the GodSquad, is a faith-based organization of clergy focused on lessening neighborhood tensions and acting as a liaison between their communities and law enforcement. The GodSquad provides violence intervention, support, and wraparound services for families impacted by violence in the East Flatbush section of Brooklyn. The work of the GodSquad also includes the establishment of Clergy for Safe

Cities (CSC), a national coalition that supports clergy-based gun violence prevention initiatives and implements a collective, comprehensive, community initiative to decrease the involvement of young people in crime and gun violence in their cities. The CSC has trained five hundred faith leaders on successful clergy-based models and best practices. For more information, see 67clergy-council.org.

BUFFALO RISING AGAINST VIOLENCE

Erie County Medical Center (ECMC) is the only major public hospital in Buffalo, New York, and the hospital where I worked the majority of my time during medical school. It also happens to be the largest trauma center in western New York, caring for high numbers of patients who are victims and survivors of violence. Buffalo Rising Against Violence (BRAVE), located at ECMC, is the region's only hospital-based violence intervention program and works alongside the community-based violence intervention program Buffalo SNUG, which stands for Should Never Use Guns and is also the word *guns* spelled backward. The BRAVE program network and Buffalo SNUG provide multifaceted intervention services that include crisis management and support, safety planning, legal services, mental health counseling, case management, job training, and linkage to substance abuse services, to name a few. For more information, see ecmc.edu/about-ecmc/brave-program.

BROWNSVILLE IN VIOLENCE OUT

Brownsville In Violence Out (BIVO) is an anti–gun violence initiative serving the 73rd Precinct of the Brownsville section of Brooklyn and is a part of the city's Crisis Management System. BIVO supports community participants between the ages of sixteen and twenty-five with a variety of services, including job training programs, access to employment, legal and therapeutic services, and school conflict mediation. BIVO is a program of the long-standing Brooklyn community-based organization CAMBA. BIVO follows the evidence-based public health Cure Violence model, which seeks to identify violently injured youth at risk for retaliatory gun violence. For more information, see camba.org/programs/brownsville-in-violence-out.

EAST FLATBUSH VILLAGE

Founded by Eric Waterman and his wife, Monique Chandler-Waterman, a community advocate and New York State Assembly member, East Flatbush Village (EFV) is an organization located in the East Flatbush section of Brooklyn dedicated to providing youth services to combat community violence. They provide programs focusing on arts, sports, financial literacy, and violence intervention. Their EFV ENOUGH (Educating Neighborhoods Organizing the Undeserved with Grassroots Organizing Healthy Initiatives) incorporates community activism through various marches, workshops, and services, some of which include Know Your Rights forums, Occupy the Corner, and Shooting Responses with their team, where they coordinate with local clergy, violence interrupters, and local elected officials to provide assistance to families impacted by gang or street violence. EFV ENOUGH has after-school programs aimed at youths aged eleven to eighteen, who have displayed conduct consistent with involvement in gang activities and other types of unproductive behavior. The goal of this program is to impact the lives of these students in a positive way, encourage them to correct their behavior, and give them necessary tools and opportunity to mentor others. For more information, see eastflatbushvillage.org.

COMMON JUSTICE

The intersecting thread among trauma, violence, and incarceration runs deep. Founded by my friend and long-term youth community servant Danielle Sered, Common Justice is "the first alternative-to-incarceration and victim-service program in the US that focuses on violent felonies in the adult courts."[3] Their work is much more than a way to divert community members from the prison system but rather an approach to "advance racial equity," address the contributors of trauma leading to incarceration, some of which include meeting with both victims and perpetrators of the crime, and provide support through their services

and partnerships. Although Common Justice is based in Brooklyn, their work is nationwide. For more information, see com
monjustice.org.

Thankfully, there are more programs like these all across the nation, and their numbers and effectiveness are constantly growing.
I hope you will be inspired to check out some of these organizations and others in your own neighborhood. We all need to
be part of the movement to address the disease of violence and
to be part of the cure.

ACKNOWLEDGMENTS

Writing this book, revisiting old journal entries, finding ideas and thoughts scribbled on random pieces of paper, and even the revolutionary act of being still to think and remember stories have all been part of my personal therapy, and I am thankful for the opportunity and the space to be able to do so. Our traumas will forever haunt us unless we take the time to process them.

There have been a great number of people who have been a part of my life, helping me to address violence, trauma, health, and healing and helping me to share this story. Meeting these people—no matter how short or how long we've known each other, whether our encounter was favorable or just a learning experience—has been rather serendipitous. There are also many people I've never met in person, some whose names I've never known, who have prayed for me, sent healing energy and encouragement, and supported KAVI and our efforts to help heal communities from trauma and violence. I want to personally thank them.

There are more than a few people I would like to thank for making this book physically and digitally possible and who supported our special movement behind the scenes.

Martha Southgate, thank you for being a most incredible collaborative writer and helping me link stories and ideas in a more palatable way. I appreciate you and your support and am already thinking about what we can do next.

Noah Daly, you believed in this project from the start and have been a motivation every step of the way. Thank you for being my writing coach, training partner, and idea builder. Love you, bruh!

Helene Atwan, thank you for being my editor and guide for this book journey and for being open to ideas that might not have been initially apparent. Your patience is legendary. I appreciate you and the team from Beacon Press, helping share our work with the world.

Regina Brooks, thank you for being my literary agent, supporting and helping to morph ideas about community, health, and trauma that could be shared with the rest of the world. You and your team from Serendipity Literary Agency have been incredible. Thank you for believing in the book's vision from early on.

Thank you to my special friends who have reviewed book chapters, helped me sort out ideas, and connect greater dots while accommodating my wayward and unnatural sleep cycle and work schedule: Tony Clark, Barnabas Crosby, Kenneth Montgomery Esq., Jason Green, Brandi Seymour, Leland Melvin, Cyndi Stivers, jessica Care moore, and Devon "Spragga" James. I can't thank you enough.

My family on the mats: Erik Nicholson, Shannon Greer, PJ Bekanich, Kwadwo Gyasi Nkita-Mayala, Frank Tornetti, Garry St. Leger, Fabio Coelho, Alessandro Bandeira, Arthan Bandeira, Gregor Gracie, my Gregor Gracie Brazilian jiu-jitsu crew, Kano Martial Arts crew, BBJJ crew, the Grappling Club, City Poly BJJ, and the RGFA crew. Thank you for your support and the lessons. I had no idea you could learn a lot from being choked, lol. But seriously, thank you for helping me better learn and practice patience, grit, and perseverance through the most gentle art and gentle way. Oss.

To my KAVI family, both past and present, and supporters, Jordan Pierre, Josiah Dobson, Terrence Francis, Rohan Walker, Melissa Elliott, Desmond McCollough, Jamal Trotman, and Kelley Cunningham, namaste.

Jacquel Clemmons-Moore, thank you for being our champion and making magic happen, Banghee Chi, Anthony Buissereth, Ramik Williams, Leander Walston, Mykhal Benjamin, Zane Patton, Dane Hall, Laetitia Brutus, Deb Ugo-Omeukwa, Chynah Jones,

Nerma LaFrance, Omarion Fanus, Keith Hill, Robert Dawson, Chanyce Taylor, Tendaji Bailey, Caleb Wright, Yahsef Johnson, Rahel Araya, Jenne Richardson, Brandon Tucker, Sherah Liverpool Archer, Bailey Ekness, Olavé Sebastien, Chanell Douglass, Courtney Cook, Taisha Smith, Natasha Nelson, Bennie Johnson, Ikim Brown, Abdul Pullium, George Hill, Anthony Carter, Tina Alston, Arkeda Hansen, Nathan Aguilar, Javaun Tomlin, Angelisa Rimondi, Jerome Louison, Shavarn Johnson, Taylor Barbuto, Ife Abdus-Salam, Azeez Alimi, Andrew Joseph Hanley, Dr. Dareema Jenkins-Hughes, Dr. Aisha Mays, Shareena Soutar, Elizabeth Ige, Dr. LeConte Dill, Jason Grant, Steve Baldi, Bro. Karim Johnson, Rahman Bugg, Ashley Ellis, Dr. Ireen Ahmed, Dr. Carla Sterling, Abena Amory-Powell, Dr. Ben Shuldiner, Dr. Ray Austin, Dr. Judie LaRosa, Dr. Keith Africa White, Dr. Robin Hayes, Dr. Scott Gassman, Janelle Ferris, Tori Lucas, Dwayne Bentley, Gene Johnson, Taagen Swaby, Franz Mullings, Kevin Harry, Corey Jeffers, Sean Rice, Dr. Muhammed-Rilwan Muritala, Rose Mitchell, Helsie Barthelus, Roderick Jenkins, Sarah Abraham, Sarah Kornhauser, Rachel Mickenburg, HSPS staff and teachers, the Eagle Academy Ocean Hill staff and teachers, School for Human Rights staff and teachers, School for Democracy and Leadership team, Wallace Niles, Marcus Holman, Rashad Meade, Takada Walls, Shaquasha Shannon, Dr. Desmond Patton, the SUNY Downstate School of Public Health, Dr. Amy Afable, Dr. Michael Joseph, Dr. Tonya Taylor, MMSEM students, Angela Lyles, Tamiru Mammo, Joe Schick, Kathy Diaz, Erik Cliette, Ny Whittaker, Tony Queseda, Emily Contillo, Jessica Mofield, Eric Cumberbatch, Dr. Sarah Jamison, Dr. Ernesto Romo, Dr. Adrienne Stevenson, Dr. Michelle Garrido, Dr. Tolu Olade, Dr. Maurice Selby, Dr. Alex Cano, Dr. Christine Ibrahim, KB Singh, Anmol Singh, Dr. Sarah Jones, Askia Askari, Anne Herrmann, Rev. Winnie Varghese, Tanya Dwyer, Rick Smith, April Glad, Flo Weiner, Lauren Glant, Kenneth Edwards, Darnell Cooper, Nona Faustine, Qiana Mestrich, Kemar James, Kema Johnson, Arthur Kirilov, Ahmed El Sayed, Devonnte Newton, Jordany Jean, Qyaji Amory-Narcisse, Carlos Cully, Lady Black, Serrina Templeman, Jude Bonney, Brandon March, Mouhamed Boureima, Dashawn Gill, and Migel Haynes.

Thank you to my friends, comrades, colleagues, mentors, and supporters who tirelessly continue to give of themselves and do vital work with our communities: Dr. Thea James, Dr. Cheryl Heron, Dr. Lynne Holden, Dr. Lynne Richardson, Dr. Sandy Scott, Dr. John Rich, Dr. Ted Corbin, Dr. Arthur Kellerman, Bro. AT Mitchell, Bro. Tislam, Bro. Dawud Mann, Dr. Carnell Cooper, Erica Ford, Bro. James Peterson, Allen James, Sis. Minyarn Johnson, Sis. Ife Charles, Amy Ellenbogen, K Bain, Marlon Peterson, Dr. Nadia Lopez, Kenton Kirby, Phil Shung, Mali X, Jazz Joseph, Dr. Princess Fortin, Clifford Larochel, Kenton Kirby, Dr. Chris Emdin, James "Jimbo" Dobbins, Dedric "Beloved" Hammond, Dr. Chris St. Vil, Paula Kovanic-Spiro, Jen Briton, Dr. Tim Murphy, Dr. David Milling, Dr. Tim McDaniel, Pastor Gil Monrose, LeVon Stone, Jumaane Williams, Stefani Zinerman, Laurie Cumbo, Diana Richardson, Tai Allen, Rob Cornegy, Zelnor Myrie, Derrick Scott, Shanduke McPhatter, Rudy Suggs, Dr. Steve Bowman, Dr. Esther Choo, Dr. Megan Ranney, Dr. Jason Prystowsky, Saba Debesu, Danielle Frilando, Danielle Thomas, Susan Cameron, Sa'uda Dunlap, Lizzie Dewan, Marlon Rice, Dr. Dumi R. L'Heureux Lewis-McCoy, Monique Chandler-Waterman, Dr. Jordan Dow, Danielle Sered, Sarah Zeller-Berkman, Dr. Roger Mitchell, Camara Jackson, Elizabeth Hayles, Dr. Abdullah Pratt, Cherie Pugh, Nina Barrett, Bishara Wilson, Hank Willis Thomas, Heidi Schwa, Jim St. Germain, Rev. Alfonso Wyatt, Dr. Michael McGee, Dr. Rueben Rutland, Dr. Keesandra Agenor, Quentin Walcott, Lacy Austin, Baz Dressinger, Dr. Donald Grant, Dr. Brigette Alexander, Dr. MJ Murphy, Dr. Juliana Jaramillo, Dr. Harry Nonez, Dr. Shawn Gibson, Jordan Canon, Hannan Sirak, Melissa Binns, Dr. Aletha Maybank, Dr. Torian Kwame Easterling, Dr. Uché Blackstock, Dr. Dara Kass, Dr. Answorth Allen, Fatima Ashraf, Kaberi Banerjee Murthy, Cecilia Clarke, Christine Hollingsworth, Shannah Dalton, Esq., Dr. Simon Fitzgerald, Dr. Melvin Stone, Dr. Valery Roudnitsky, Dr. Leon Boudourakis, Dr. Tim Schwartz, Dr. Asher Hirshberg, Dr. Audrey Sealey, Jessica Gamzon, Tony Welters, Deborah Sealy, Mattie Singh, Linnea Ashley, Anne Marks, Dr. Ambreen Khan, Dr. Sigrid Wolfram, Dr. Jessica Stetz, Dr. Donald Doukas, Dr. Mark Silverberg, Dr. Joshua McHugh, Dr. Krystle Johnson, Dr.

James Hassel, Dr. Alex Brevil, Fred Harry, Tracey Bagley, Sandra Guzman, Tamara Houston, Dr. Tyeese Gaines, Natasha Gaspard, Alice Blair, Dr. Bonnie Baron, Dr. Italo Brown, Deiniol Buxton, Dr. Endy Cadet, Dr. Jonel Daphnis, Dr. Emily Nichols, Dr. Markus Little, Dr. Kelly Maurelus, Dr. Kareen Thompson, Dr. Karen Staville, Dr. Ian deSouza, Dr. James Willis, Rebecca Fisher, Shaina Harrison, Leticia Theodore-Green, Michelle Genece Patterson, Kathleen Toner, David Gonzalez, Dr. Alden Landry, Dr. Louis Rolston-Cregler, Dr. Sheldon Tepperman, Adele Flateau, Debra Tyndall, Rita Joseph, Dr. Brooke Learner, Dr. Ron Moscati, Sheldon McLeod, Faye Mitchell, Alexis Davis, Seth Narine, Graham Gulian, Donovan Vassell, Dawn Walker, Sarah Abraham, Dr. Michael Lucchesi, Dr. Rajesh Verma, Dr. Elias Youssef, Dr. Brittany Choe, Dr. Andrew Sweeny, Lashawn Peña, Martha Patella, Dr. Wendy Lau, Dr. Christiana Sim, Dr. Ninfa Mehta, Dr. Roger Holt, Dr. Ric Leno, Dr. Chris Doty, Dr. Selwena Brewster, Kings County–SUNY Downstate Department of Emergency Medicine, Kings County Hospital Department of Trauma, Kings County Hospital Center staff, Dr. Brian McNeil, Dr. Teresa Smith, Dr. Carla Boutin Foster, Dr. Anika Daniels-Osaze, Tony Martin, Sheri Howard, Ingrid Browne, Cook County Hospital Department of Emergency Medicine, Cook County Hospital Department of Trauma, EMEDEX, Dr. Stephan Rinnert, Dr. Christina Bloem, Dr. Bonnie Arquilla, Patricia Roblin, the Arthur Ashe Institute, the Wakandans, Presidential Leadership Scholars, TED Res, CNN Heroes, Black & TED, Mike Hettwer, Henry Goodgame, Dr. Illya Davis, Curtis Valentine, Cynthia Charles, Caron Scott, Dr. Hope Tait, Dr. Camilo Galeano Londono, Rev. C. Vernon Mason, and the Costagliola-Teatum Family.

To my family and friends: I might not call you back right away, or respond to text messages for weeks, but I am grateful for you all.

Special thanks to the Gore Family, Curry Family, Frazier Family, Bouvia Family, Long Family, Sturdivant Family, Yvonne Curry, Richard Tucker, Sheila Anderson, Russell Frederick, Bayeté Ross Smith, Dr. Ramon Gist, Seth Byrd, Derick Petersen, Brian "Deka" Paupaw, Dr. Ché Ward, Dr. Troy Abernathy, Michael Coppock, Esq., Dr. Antonio Graham, Kwane Andrews, Dr. Eric Tait,

Dr. Lauren Smith, Dr. Trevonne Thompson, Matt Fields, Dr. Joseph Feagan, Dr. Aisha Holder, Uwa Aghedo, the Browne Family, Wheeler Family, Yeshi TimKee, Issa Aiko Lalibela Fabrega, Erin Stevens, Luz Salazar, the Solomon Family, Legesse Family, Linda Young and family, Berry Rice, the Clouden Family, Gardner Family, Banyan Family, Bruno Family, Reilly Family, Lister Family, Sara Ayele, Jethro Waters, Nigat Ayele, Rahel Getachew, Maro Haile, G. Desta, Janan Rajalingam, Hannah Rajalingam, Helena Rajalingam, Jessica Maldonado, Jalia Maldonado, Dr. Jane Kim, Dr. Randi Burlew, Antoinette Campbell, Alex Merceron, Tamara Hood, Shannon Washington, Jessica Chong, Kellie Cole, Simeon Sessley, the Knox-Houchens Family, Walters-deFreitas Family, Cynthia Charles, Shani Jamila, Malikha Mallette, and Tiffani Hutton.

My parents, Patricia Curry and Bob Gore, thank you for being my greatest teachers and guides, allowing your free-spirited child to explore the world.

To Jason Curry and Angel Maldonado—thank you for being my brothers. The lessons from you both have helped me become a man and share my gifts with others.

To my ancestral family—Grandaddy, Grandma, Brenda Tucker, Mama, Robert, Rochelle, Beverly, Brenda Sturdivant, Khandice, Legesse aka Papa Legs, and Willis Young—thank you for being guides and watching over. I miss you.

Last but not least, I want to thank my wife, Hibist Legesse, and son, Araya Gore. Thank you for loving me, for being my most important support, inspiration, and for keeping me grounded. I love you

IN REMEMBRANCE:
Willis Young, Zahara Lewis, Lavon Walker, George Harris, John Wright, Esq., Deanna Rodriguez, Esq., Rev. Dr. Calvin Butts—thank you for your light.

If I have forgotten to mention anyone it wasn't because you aren't in my heart. I blame it 100 percent on sleep deprivation. Thank you for understanding.

NOTES

INTRODUCTION: CONFRONTING VIOLENCE

1. R. Gore, *Healing Inner City Trauma* (video), TED Talk, New York City, July 2016, https://www.ted.com/talks/rob_gore_healing_inner_city _trauma.

2. M. Heron, "Deaths: Leading Causes for 2018," *National Vital Statistics Reports* 70, no. 4 (2021).

3. City of New York, "NYPD Announces November Crime Statistics," news release, December 8, 2021, https://www.nyc.gov/site/nypd/news/pr1208 /nypd-november-crime-statistics.

4. W. Li, C. Onyebeke, M. Huynh, A. Castro, L. Falci, S. Gurung, D. Levy, J. Kennedy, G. Maduro, Y. Sun, S. Evergreen, and G. Van Wye, *Summary of Vital Statistics*, Bureau of Vital Statistics, New York City Department of Health and Mental Hygiene, 2019, https://www.nyc.gov/assets /doh/downloads/pdf/vs/2019sum.pdf.

5. US Census Bureau, "New York State Population Topped 20 Million in 2020," July 28, 2022, https://www.census.gov/library/stories /state-by-state/new-york-population-change-between-census-decade. html; Mayor's Office of Criminal Justice, "Shooting Incidents by Borough NYC," n.d., https://criminaljustice.cityofnewyork.us/individual_charts /shooting-incident-by-borough, accessed January 11, 2023; Mayor's Office of Criminal Justice, "Violent Crime by Borough NYC," n.d., https://criminaljustice.cityofnewyork.us/individual_charts/ violent-crime-by-borough, accessed November 3, 2023.

6. K. Hinterland et al., *Brownsville: Community Health Profiles 2018*, Brooklyn Community District 16, NYC Health 40, no. 59 (2018): 1–20; K. Hinterland et al., *Crown Heights and Prospect Heights: Community Health Profiles 2018*, Brooklyn Community District 8, NYC Health 32,

no. 59 (2018): 1–20; K. Hinterland et al., *East New York and Starrett City: Community Health Profiles 2018*, Brooklyn Community District 5, NYC Health 29, no. 59 (2018): 1–20.

7. K. Hinterland et al., *East Flatbush: Community Health Profiles 2018*, Brooklyn Community District 17, NYC Health 41, no. 59 (2018): 1–20.

8. R. M. Cunningham et al., "Youth Seeking Emergency Department Care for Assault-Related Injury: A 2-Year Prospective Cohort Study," *JAMA Pediatrics* 169, no. 1 (2015): 63–70.

9. S. Saif et al., "Higher Risk of Mortality in Intentional Traumatic Injuries: A Multivariate Regression Analysis of a Trauma Registry," *Bulletin of Emergency and Trauma* 8, no. 2 (2020): 107–10.

10. S. R. Keglar et al., "Vital Signs: Changes in Firearm Homicide and Suicide Rates—United States, 2019–2020," *Morbidity and Mortality Weekly Report* 71, no. 19 (2022): 656–63.

11. N. M. Simske et al., "Implementation of Programming for Survivors of Violence-Related Trauma at a Level 1 Trauma Center," *Trauma Surgery & Acute Care Open* 6 (2021): e000739.

12. Centers for Disease Control, *The Public Health Approach to Violence Prevention*, National Center for Injury Prevention and Control, Division of Violence Prevention, n.d., https://www.cdc.gov/violenceprevention /pdf/PH_App_Violence-a.pdf, accessed January 15, 2023.

CHAPTER 1: LOSING WILLIS

1. Caught in the Crossfire is the first hospital-based violence intervention program in the US and is part of the Youth ALIVE! nonprofit, based in Oakland, California. This was the first violence intervention program I'd ever read about, and its organization helped spark the development of what eventually became KAVI. See https://www.youthalive.org.

2. SOS, a program under the Center for Court Innovation, is dedicated to ending "gun violence at the neighborhood level by changing lo-cal norms around violence and creating opportunities for meaningful educational and employment opportunities within the community," according to their website. See https://www.courtinnovation.org/pro grams/save-our-streets-sos for more information. Man Up! Inc. is a community-based nonprofit in Brooklyn, New York, dedicated to pro-viding services for neighborhood improvement. Some of these services include violence intervention and interruption, youth programming, and job training. See http://manupinc.org for more information.

3. VIAP at Boston Medical Center was founded in 2006 to provide support for victims and survivors of intentional violence in the Greater Boston area. It was founded by a mentor of mine, Dr. Thea James, who gave me my first exposure to emergency medicine when I was a college student. See https://www.bmc.org/violence-intervention-advocacy-program.

CHAPTER 2: JUMPED

1. K. Kozlowska et al., "Fear and the Defense Cascade: Clinical Implications and Management," *Harvard Review of Psychiatry* 23, no. 4 (July–August 2015): 263–87.

2. F. Ozbay et al., "Social Support and Resilience to Stress," *Psychiatry* 4, no. 5 (May 2007): 35–40.

3. V. J. Felitti et al., "Relationship of Childhood Abuse and Household Dysfunction to Many of the Leading Causes of Death in Adults," Adverse Childhood Experiences Study, *American Journal of Preventive Medicine* 14, no. 4 (May 1998): 245–58.

4. M. T. Merrick et al., "Vital Signs: Estimated Proportion of Adult Health Problems Attributable to Adverse Childhood Experiences and Implications for Prevention—25 States, 2015–2017," *Morbidity and Mortality Weekly Report* 68 (2019): 999–1005, http://dx.doi.org/10.15585/mmwr .mm6844e1.

5. Compassion Prison Project, based in Los Angeles, is dedicated to transforming prisons from "punitive human warehouses into rehabilitative environments." See https://compassionprisonproject.org.

6. K. Ford et al., "Adverse Childhood Experiences: A Retrospective Study to Understand Their Associations with Lifetime Mental Health Diagnosis, Self-Harm or Suicide Attempt, and Current Low Mental Wellbeing in a Male Welsh Prison Population" *Health Justice* 8, no. 13 (2020), https:// doi.org/10.1186/s40352-020-00115-5.

7. N. N. Duke et al., "Adolescent Violence Perpetration: Associations with Multiple Types of Adverse Childhood Experiences," *Pediatrics* 125, no. 4 (2010): e778–e786.

CHAPTER 3: F THE POLICE

1. Jim Carnes, *Us and Them: A History of Intolerance in America* (New York: Oxford University Press, 1999).

2. "Remembering the Crown Heights Riot 25 Years On," WNYC News, August 19, 2016.

3. R. Brame et al., "Demographic Patterns of Cumulative Arrest Prevalence by Ages 18 and 23," *Crime & Delinquency* 60, no. 3 (2014): 471–86, https://doi.org/10.1177/0011128713514801.

4. Cathy J. Cohen, "Black Youth Culture Survey," Black Youth Project, Chicago, 2005, http://www.blackyouthproject.com, accessed January 19, 2023.

CHAPTER 4: GETTING ON TRACK

1. A. Elklit et al., "Childhood Maltreatment and School Problems: A Danish National Study," *Scandinavian Journal of Educational Research* 62, no. 1 (2018): 150–59; A. S. Morrow et al., "Direct and Indirect Pathways from Adverse Childhood Experiences to High School Dropout Among

High-Risk Adolescents," *Journal of Research on Adolescence* 28, no. 2 (2018): 327–41.

2. D. Finkelhor et al., "Prevalence of Childhood Exposure to Violence, Crime, and Abuse: Results from the National Survey of Children's Exposure to Violence," *JAMA Pediatrics* 169, no. 8 (2015): 746–54.

CHAPTER 5: THE SWATS, RED DOGS, AND THE REALITY OUTSIDE THE MOREHOUSE GATES

1. *Atlanta Police Department Policy Manual, Standard Operating Procedure*, APD.SOP.1010, Mission and Organization of the Department, December 10, 2010.

2. G. K. Singh and H. Lee, "Marked Disparities in Life Expectancy by Education, Poverty Level, Occupation, and Housing Tenure in the United States, 1997–2014," *International Journal of Maternal and Child Health and AIDS* 10, no. 1 (2021): 7–18.

CHAPTER 6: RUFF BUFF AND THE PRICE OF DISINVESTMENT

1. James H. Jones, *Bad Blood: The Tuskegee Syphilis Experiment* (New York: Free Press, 1981); H. A. Washington, *Medical Apartheid: The Dark History of Medical Experimentation on Black Americans from Colonial Times to the Present* (New York: Doubleday, 2006); Rebecca Skloot, *The Immortal Life of Henrietta Lacks* (New York: Crown, 2010).

2. A. L. Fairchild and R. Bayer, "Uses and Abuses of Tuskegee," *Science* 284, no. 5416 (2010): 919–21.

3. J. M. Douglas, "Penicillin Treatment of Syphilis," *JAMA* 301, no. 7 (2009): 769–71, doi:10.1001/jama.2009.143.

4. Skloot, *The Immortal Life of Henrietta Lacks*.

5. Maria Cramer, "Henrietta Lacks, Whose Cells Were Taken Without Her Consent, Is Honored by W.H.O.," *New York Times*, October 13, 2021.

6. I. Xiearli and M. Nivet, "The Racial and Ethnic Composition and Distribution of Primary Care Physicians," *Journal of Health Care for the Poor and Underserved* 29, no. 1 (2018): 556–70.

7. US Department of Health and Human Services, Office of Disease Prevention and Health Promotion, *Healthy People 2030*, https://health.gov/healthypeople, accessed May 31, 2023.

CHAPTER 7: TO TREAT SUFFERING, KNOW SUFFERING

1. Frantz Fanon, *The Wretched of the Earth* (New York: Penguin, 1967).

2. E. Heath, "Berlin Conference of 1884–1885," in *Encyclopedia of Africa*, ed. Kwame Anthony Appiah and Henry Louis Gates Jr. (New York: Oxford University Press, 2010).

3. World Health Organization, "Health Workforce Requirements for

Universal Health Coverage and the Sustainable Development Goals," background paper no. 1, Global Strategy on Human Resources for Health, 2016.

4. "Mortality and Causes of Death Collaborators Global, Regional, and National Age-Sex Specific All-Cause and Cause-Specific Mortality for 240 Causes of Death, 1990–2013: A Systematic Analysis for the Global Burden of Disease Study 2013," *Lancet* 385, no. 9963 (2015): 117–71.

CHAPTER 8: SOMETHING EXCITING

1. David Ansell, *County: Life, Death and Politics at Chicago's Public Hospital* (Chicago: Academy Chicago Publishers, 2012).

2. Steven D. Levitt and Stephen J. Dubner, *Freakonomics* (New York: Harper Trophy, 2006).

3. J. A. Rich and C. M. Grey, "Pathways to Recurrent Trauma Among Young Black Men: Traumatic Stress, Substance Use, and the 'Code of the Street,'" *American Journal of Public Health* 95, no. 5 (May 2005): 816–24.

4. C. Delgado, "Making a Difference: An Interview with Sherman Spears," *Colorlines*, December 15, 1998, https://colorlines.com/article/making-difference-interview-sherman-spears.

5. Youth Alive!, "Our Mission," n.d., https://www.youthalive.org/about, accessed January 22, 2023.

6. P. D. Gatseva and M. Argirova, "Public Health: The Science of Promoting Health," *Journal of Public Health* 19, no. 3 (2011): 205–6.

7. National Center for Injury and Prevention Control, "Youth Violence: Fact Sheet," 2003, http://www.cdc.gov/ncipc/factsheets/yvfacts.htm.

8. Elijah Anderson, *Code of the Street: Decency, Violence, and the Moral Life of the Inner City* (New York: W. W. Norton & Co., 1999).

9. Kurt R. Denninghoff et al., "Emergency Medicine: Competencies for Youth Violence Prevention and Control," *Academic Emergency Medicine* 9, no. 9 (2002): 947–56.

CHAPTER 9: THE PIPELINE

1. Association of American Medical Colleges, *Altering the Course: Black Males in Medicine*, report, Washington, DC, 2015.

2. Brian D. Smedley, Adrienne Y. Stith, Lois Colburn, and Clyde H. Evans, *The Right Thing to Do, The Smart Thing to Do: Enhancing Diversity in the Health Professions*, summary of the symposium on diversity in health professions in honor of Herbert W. Nickens, MD, Institute of Medicine (Washington, DC: National Academies Press, 2001).

CHAPTER 11: DO SOMETHING

1. H. M. Sheet, "In Portland, Falling Stars Shine a Light on Gun Violence: A Personal Loss, in Part, Drives Artist Hank Willis Thomas to Confront One

of the Biggest Fears Among African-American Men," *New York Times*, October 23, 2019.

2. Question Bridge, "About Question Bridge," n.d., http://questionbridge .com, accessed January 22, 2023.

3. Alex Kotlowitz, "Blocking the Transmission of Violence," *New York Times Magazine*, May 4, 2008.

4. R. W. Kelly, *Crime and Enforcement Activity in New York City*, New York Police Department, 2011, https://www.nyc.gov/assets/nypd/down loads/pdf/analysis_and_planning/yearend2011enforcementreport.pdf.

CHAPTER 12: THE MANY FACES OF VIOLENCE

1. Frank Herbert, *Dune* (orig. 1965; New York: Ace Books, 2005).

2. K. N. Deering et al., "A Systematic Review of the Correlates of Violence Against Sex Workers," *American Journal of Public Health* 104, no. 5 (May 2014): e42–e54.

3. A. L. Wirtz et al., "Gender-Based Violence Against Transgender People in the United States: A Call for Research and Programming," *Trauma, Violence & Abuse* 21, no. 2 (2020): 227–41.

4. K. I. Fredriksen et al., "Health, Economic and Social Disparities Among Transgender Women, Transgender Men and Transgender Nonbinary Adults: Results from a Population-Based Study," *Preventive Medicine* 156 (2022): 106988.

5. L. Langenderfer-Magruder et al., "Sexual Victimization and Subsequent Police Reporting by Gender Identity Among Lesbian, Gay, Bisexual, Transgender, and Queer Adults," *Violence and Victims* 31, no. 2 (2016): 320–31.

6. A. O. Gyamerah et al., "Experiences and Factors Associated with Trans-phobic Hate Crimes Among Transgender Women in the San Fran-cisco Bay Area: Comparisons Across Race," *BMC Public Health* 21 (2021): 1053.

7. M. J. Breiding et al., *Intimate Partner Violence Surveillance: Uniform Definitions and Recommended Data Elements, Version 2.0*, Atlanta: National Center for Injury Prevention and Control, Centers for Disease Control and Prevention, 2015.

8. R. W. Leemis et al., *National Intimate Partner and Sexual Violence Sur-vey: 2016/17*, report on Intimate Partner Violence, Atlanta: Centers for Disease Control and Prevention, 2022, https://www.cdc.gov/violencepre vention/pdf/nisvs/nisvsreportonipv_2022.pdf.

9. US Preventive Service Task Force, "Screening for Intimate Partner Vi-olence, Elder Abuse, and Abuse of Vulnerable Adults: Recommendation Statement," *American Family Physician* 99, no. 10 (2019). Consciously screening for partner violence leads to early identification of the problem, with the goal of mobilizing resources to provide the greatest level of sup-

port for the survivor. There are a series of different screening tools that can be of help, but the following are some that have been recommended by the US Preventive Service Task Force: Humiliation, Afraid, Rape, Kick (HARK); Hurt, Insult, Threaten, Scream (HITS); Extended - Hurt, Insult, Threaten, Scream (E-HITS); Partner Violence Screening (PVS) tool; and Woman Abuse Screening Tool (WAST). I do not endorse any particular tool but have more experience using the HITS screening. The screenings mentioned above, with each method comprising a unique set of three to eight questions that can be easily asked in a private setting. Screening is only a small fraction of the intervention process. Interventions that are most effective at decreasing the short- and long-term consequences of partner violence incorporate regular counseling, home support, and parental support and address multiple risk factors.

10. NYC Health and Hospitals/Kings County, "NYC Health + Hospitals/ Kings County Launches a Clinical Forensic Medicine Fellowship," news release, July 6, 2022, http://clinicalmonster.com/wp-content /uploads/2022/07/KCH-Forensic-Fellowship.pdf.

CHAPTER 13: THE KAVI WAY

1. High School for Public Service website, https://www.highschoolforpublic service.com.
2. Pauline W. Chen, "Breaking the Cycle of Violence," *New York Times*, January 13, 2011.
3. *Trauma and Treatment: How Violence Interrupters Help Heal*, J. Lief, prod., and A. Maldonado, dir., 2022, retrieved from YouTube, https://www .youtube.com/watch?v=4iDTPtCc-GM.
4. Elizabeth Kübler-Ross, *On Death and Dying* (New York: Collier Books/ Macmillan, 1970).

CHAPTER 14: IN HONOR OF WILLIS

1. E. Grinshteyn and D. Hemenway, "Violent Death Rates: The US Compared with Other High-Income OECD Countries," *American Journal of Medicine* 129, no. 3 (March 2016): 266–73.
2. J. Holt-Lunstad et al., "Social Relationships and Mortality Risk: A Meta-Analytic Review," *PLOS Medicine* 7, no. 7 (2010): e1000316.
3. B. Adini et al., "Earlier Detection of Public Health Risks–Health Policy Lessons for Better Compliance with the International Health Regulations (IHR 2005): Insights from Low-, Mid- and High-Income Countries," *Health Policy* (Amsterdam) 123, no. 10 (2019): 941–46.
4. A. Biglan et al., "The Critical Role of Nurturing Environments for Promoting Human Well-Being," *American Psychologist* 67, no. 4 (2012): 257–71.

CONCLUSION: RESOURCES FOR VIOLENCE PREVENTION AND TREATMENT

1.   S. Levine et al., "Health Care Industry Insights: Why the Use of Preventive Services Is Still Low," *Preventing Chronic Disease* 16 (2019), https://doi.org/10.5888/pcd16.180625.

2.   C. Juillard et al., "Saving Lives and Saving Money: Hospital-Based Violence Intervention Is Cost-Effective," *Journal of Trauma and Acute Care Surgery* 78 (2015): 252–58.

3.   Common Justice, "Our Work," n.d., https://www.commonjustice.org/our_work, accessed March 31, 2023.